DATE DUE

Essays in Social Neuroscience

Essays in Social Neuroscience

edited by John T. Cacioppo and Gary G. Berntson

A Bradford Book
The MIT Press
Cambridge, Massachusetts
London, England

This book was set in Stone Serif and Stone Sans by SNP Best-set Typesetter Ltd., Hong Kong.
Printed and bound in the United States of America.

Library of Congress Cataloging-in-Publication Data

Essays in social neuroscience / edited by John T. Cacioppo, Gary G. Berntson.
    p. cm.—(Social neuroscience series)
"A Bradford book."
ISBN 0-262-03323-2 (alk. paper)
1. Neurosciences—Social aspects.   2. Psychoneuroendocrinology.
I. Cacioppo, John T.   II. Berntson, Gary G.   III. Series.

RC343.E876 2004
612.8—dc22   2003070605

10 9 8 7 6 5 4 3 2 1

Contents

Preface

Before the Enlightenment, most people neither read nor wrote, human productivity was not much higher than it had been for thousands of years, and the average person lived in conditions that, by contemporary standards, would be considered squalid. In contrast, the twentieth century was a period of unparalleled advance in science, when even the human mind attracted serious scientific attention.

To simplify the study of the mind, neuroscientists in the past century tended to ignore or hold constant social influences, while cognitive and social scientists tended to ignore the biological constraints on and mechanisms through which cognition, affect, and conation are expressed. As conceived by the neurosciences, the architects of development and behavior were anatomical structures and genetic strings sculpted by the forces of evolution operating over millennia and encapsulated within living cells far from the reach of social influences; the brain was an analytical information-processing machine. Information attributable to the social world, the reasoning often went, was best considered later, if and when the need arose; social factors were thought to have minimal implications for basic development, structure, or processes of the brain or mind, and thus to be essentially irrelevant. But even if social factors proved relevant, considering them may render the study of the human mind and behavior too complicated to sustain scientific progress.

The century's two world wars, Great Depression, and widespread civil injustices made it amply clear, however, that social and cultural forces were too important to await the full explication of cellular and molecular mechanisms. Thus cognitive and social scientists alike came to ignore biological constraints, mechanisms, and insights, often with the misguided intention of protecting the behavioral sciences from the onslaught of reductionism. A systematic approach to investigating the parts to better understand the whole, reductionism is sometimes confused with substitutionism (replacing a higher level, such as social representation, with a lower level, such as cellular representation). Reductionism uses data derived from distinct levels of analysis to both constrain and inspire the interpretation of data derived from other levels of analysis. In reductionism, the whole is as important as the parts, for only in examining the interplay across levels of analysis can the design of the whole be ascertained. Indeed, more than three centuries ago, Nicolaus Steno observed that "the brain is a machine. . . . There remains to be done, therefore, only what would be done for all other machines. I mean the dismantling of all its components, piece by piece, and consideration of what they can do separately and as a whole" (Steno, 1669).

In fairness, the specialized knowledge and fundamental research that were required to cultivate descriptive taxonomies, theoretical formulations, and methodologies—coupled with an early emphasis on isolated scientific work—all but ensured that social and biological perspectives would be developed in isolation from each other.

In the twilight of the twentieth century, united in their common view that information processing could best be understood by appeal to both the brain and its emergent manifestation, the mind, and in their common goal of understanding how the mind works, neuroscientists and cognitive scientists began to collaborate more systematically. These collaborations have helped unravel puzzles of the mind, in particular, aspects of perception, imagery, attention, and memory. Many other such puzzles, however, require a more comprehensive approach to the mystery of mind-brain connections and mind-body orchestration, puzzles such as attraction, altruism, affiliation, attachment, attitudes, identification, kin recognition, communication, cooperation, competition, commerce, empathy, sexuality, communication, dominance, persuasion, obedience, morality, contagion, love, nurturance, violence, and person memory, to name the most notable.

As the twenty-first century dawns, there is a recognition that much of the groundwork for multidisciplinary scientific collaborations has been laid by the giants of the preceding three centuries. Neuroscientists, cognitive scientists, and social scientists are placing less emphasis on the arbitrary division between the social and the biological sciences and are moving beyond simplifying assumptions toward developing more comprehensive theories of mind, brain, biology, and behavior. Through the efforts of such individuals and the interests of an increasing number of graduate and postdoctoral trainees, the broad multidisciplinary perspective of social neuroscience has emerged.

These essays tell the story of some of the major leaders in social neuroscience. The range of disciplines and questions they address, from genetics to social structures, speaks volumes about the breadth and potential of the social neuroscience perspective. The essays also illustrate that, although individual scientists must make trade-offs between breadth and depth of expertise, the broader scientific community can lessen if not eliminate the costs of such trade-offs through collective interdisciplinary efforts—which is itself a kind of emergent property.

The contributors were asked to briefly introduce readers to their perspectives on and research in social neuroscience; to indicate why the big questions addressed in their research are worthwhile questions regarding human mind and behavior; and to tie discussion of the various facets of their research to their unique perspective on, and contributions to, the field. Because a hallmark of social neuroscience is the use of multiple methods, often bridging multiple levels of analysis, the contributors were further encouraged to discuss which specific questions required which specific methodologies and levels of analysis, and why multiple methodologies and multiple levels of analysis proved helpful. Moreover, they were asked to avoid the extensive use of technical terms and citations of the work of others typical of scholarly presentations so that readers might better understand the theoretical frameworks guiding the contributors' research and might be more likely to enjoy and learn from reading essays about research pursuits distant from their own interests.

Work on this volume was funded by a grant BCS-0086314 from the National Science Foundation, an institution that has long and tirelessly supported efforts to bridge the divide between the social, cognitive, and neurosciences. Our thanks go to Tom Stone at the MIT Press for his invaluable support and to our coeditors from Foundations in Social Neuroscience series, themselves contributors to the current volume, for their unfailing expertise and support. To have friends and colleagues who are also such brilliant and generous scientists is a gift we cherish. We hope readers will enjoy reading about their fascinating research, and learning more about social neuroscience and its potential in the century ahead.

Reference

Steno, N. (1669). Cited on p. 1 of Swanson, L. W. (2003). *Brain architecture*. New York: Oxford University Press.

Essays in Social Neuroscience

1 The Nature of Nurture: Maternal Effects and Chromatin Remodeling

Michael J. Meaney

My Life in Science as a John Mellencamp Song

Considering the developmental focus of the work undertaken by my colleagues and me, it seems appropriate to begin with some reference to my own academic, early experience. I began my life in science under the tutelage of Professor Jane Stewart, a preeminent behavioral neuroscientist. One can do no better. I have never really understood what was meant by the word *instinct*. An action repeated effortlessly, immutable in form, unerring in consequence? Jane's ability to mentor research fellows was such. I believe she is without peer. Jane was married to Dalbir Bindra, perhaps the leading theorist in psychology of his day. D.B., as he was called, was a titan of dignity, charm, and intellectual generosity. To my great fortune, D.B. had a bad back that precluded shoveling snow. And it snows considerably in Montreal. Thus it came to pass, that following any significant snowfall, we would, appropriately enough, ascend the hill to where Jane and D.B. lived, and clear the driveway. Our reward was to then breakfast with Jane and D.B. on eggs, juice, and a discussion of the most recent version of a chapter of D.B.'s book. I love snowfalls in ways that no one else can ever appreciate.

Following my doctoral studies, I moved to the the Rockefeller University and the laboratory of Professor Bruce McEwen. I suspect there are few who will read this without having some impression of Bruce's remarkable reputation for excellence in science and mentorship. It is all well deserved. There is little good in my career that has not in some way been derived from my sojourn in Bruce's lab.

The parenting was thus sublime. And in the midst of all this was I, focused from my earliest days as an undergraduate on precisely the same scientific interest, the biology of individual differences. For an offspring of Montreal, the home of Hans Selye and Donald Hebb, my studies of the development of individual differences in endocrine responses to stress seem as if destiny. I fell in love with this topic as a sophomore. My affection has never wavered. Scientifically, I married my childhood sweetheart. I still live in my hometown. And I yearn to transmit to mine what was bestowed upon me. Actually, it has all been rather simple.

You Can't Get There from Here

Following a public lecture, a journalist approached the renowned psychologist Donald Hebb and asked for his opinion on which contributed more to personality, nature or nurture. Hebb responded that this was akin to asking what contributed more to the area of a rectangle, the length or the width. Like all good urban myths, there are multiple versions of this story. The context changes somewhat, but Hebb's reply remains intact in its piercing brilliance. Forty some years later, we pace about in the same state of confusion, pondering the same foolish question, armed with the impressive tools of a new millennium, but without the wisdom of Hebb.

We have ample reason to celebrate the advances associated with the human genome project, yet the same technology bears the risk of expanding the divide between the biological and social sciences. One group of scientists is blindly infatuated with the explanations derived from gene sequencing consortiums; the other huddles in fear at the thought of a biological maze in which it is lost. Such divisions, by definition, only further confuse the study of development as scientists from different disciplines retreat further into their respect comfort zones. Can you imagine the study of "rectangularity" composed of those who study "lengths" and those who study "widths"? Ultimately, one would hope, individuals would emerge demanding an integrative approach that recognizes only the study of rectangles, dismissing the notion that anything meaningful can come from the study of "lengths" or "widths" alone. Such an advance would require no new tools, but rather a change in the way we think about rectangles.

Life does not emerge as a function of either nature or nurture. And it is equally wrong to assume that phenotype derives from *both* nature *and* nurture. For this is only to repeat the misunderstanding in kinder, gentler terms. Both conclusions are derived from additive models of determinism where gene + environment = phenotype. Such models make no biological sense whatsoever. To paraphrase Lewontin (1980), life emerges only from the interaction between the two: there are no genetic factors that can be studied independent of the environment, and there are no environmental factors that function independent of the genome. Phenotype emerges only from the interaction of gene and environment. Nature and nurture do not exist in a manner that can ever be considered as independently quantifiable. At no level can the function of a gene be separated from its cellular environment; it is biologically absurd to assume otherwise. Every trait is a function of the interaction between gene X and the environment. And, lest you think I am simply some environmental wolf in sheep's clothing, it is equally absurd to believe that the environmental factors can be studied independent of the genome and the constraints it places on the neural systems that serve as the inevitable bridge between environment and effect.

Dearest Mommy, Do Parents Really Matter?

My laboratory examines gene—environment interactions through studies of the effects of maternal care on gene expression and phenotypic development in mammals. The developmental outcomes involve measures of endocrine and behavioral responses to adversity, or stress. Indeed, our studies follow from a well-established theme in biology: maternal effects on the development of defensive responses to threat. Such effects are apparent in virtually all forms of life. In a remarkable paper, Agarwal, Laforsch, and Tollrian (1999) provided evidence for transgenerational, maternal effects in two models: one a plant, and the other an insect. Herbivory results in the expression of inducible defenses (defensive reactions occurring in response to specific forms of provocation) in plants. In the radish, damage from a caterpillar induces an increased production of mustard oil glycosides and a greater density of setose trichomes on newly formed leaves. These defenses protect against subsequent attacks. Plants expressing such defenses have a significantly greater lifetime seed production. And there are consequences for the next generation. The seedlings derived from the caterpillar-damaged radishes showed significant changes in glycosinolate profiles and altered trichome expression: the number of tri-chomes per leaf was increased in seedlings as a function of maternal herbivory. Only the mothers, and not the seedlings themselves, had ever been exposed to herbivory in any form. Such changes were adaptive. Caterpillars gained significantly less weight, presumably from reduced consumption, when exposed to seedlings from damaged versus undamaged mothers.

This is but one example of maternal effects. The capacity for flight in grasshoppers, the tail length of lizards, and the helmet size of water fleas are all determined by maternal effects acting through unknown mechanisms. The fundamental principle here is that of maternal regulation of the development of rudimentary defensive responses to threat. These are classic examples of epigenetic, or nongenomic, inheritance, where traits of the parents are transmitted to offspring in a manner not dependent on information encoded in the nuclear genes. Maternal effects in plants and insects alter the form and intensity of defensive responses to threat. The environmental experience of the mother is thus translated through an epigenetic mechanism of inheritance into phenotypic variation in the offspring. Indeed, maternal effects could result in the transmission of adaptive responses across generations. My colleagues and I argue that similar effects occur in mammals and are derived, in part, from variations in maternal care during postnatal life. As in nonmammalian species, these effects also target rudimentary defensive responses.

Le Rat de Ville (and the Other One)

Amazingly, a female rat commonly gives birth to a litter of 10–15 pups that, before weaning, will weigh more than she

does. Over this period, the dam remains the sole source of nutri-
ents and fluids. In a laboratory setting, lactating mother rats
vary little in the amount of time spent in physical contact with
their pups, alternating between nursing bouts with their offspring and time alone to attend to their deeply challenged metabolic equilibrium. A nursing bout commences when the mother
approaches the nest, gathers the pups underneath her ventral
surface, and licks and grooms her offspring. The licking and
grooming arouses the pups, which then vigorously attach to a
nipple and suckle. In the next minutes, there ensues a milk
letdown and a relaxation of the pups. The dam again licks the
pups, which despite being engorged with milk, scurry underneath her and compete enthusiastically for nipples in the misguided assumption that a Wisconsin dairy farm lurks only a few
millimeters down the road. This is nonnutritive suckling as
competitive sport. Over the first week of life, about 30 percent
of the maternal licking is directed toward the pups' anogenital
region. This is essential. Pups will not otherwise urinate. The
bounty for the mother lies in the ingestion of the sodium-
enriched urine.

There are highly stable individual differences in licking and
grooming (LG) such that over the first week of life some (i.e.,
high-LG) mothers consistently lick and groom their pups about
three times as frequently as do other (i.e., low-LG) mothers. This
information is gleaned from hours of observations per day of
individual mothers with their litters under perfectly undis-
turbed conditions. It is an ideal activity for long Canadian
winters.

These naturally occurring variations in maternal care are associated with individual differences in hypothalamic-pituitary-
adrenal (HPA) axis responses to stress (there are also differences

in behavioral responses to stress, but for the sake of this essay I will limit my comments to the HPA axis). As adults, the offspring of mothers that undertake frequent licking and grooming and arched-back nursing (high-LG-ABN mothers) are behaviorally less fearful and show more modest HPA responses to stress than the offspring of mothers that do not (low-LG-ABN mothers; Liu et al., 1997). Cross-fostering studies show that the biological offspring of low-LG-ABN mothers reared by high-LG-ABN dams resemble the normal offspring of high-LG-ABN (and vice versa; Francis, Dioro, Liu, & Meaney, 1999). These findings suggest that variations in maternal behavior can directly influence the development of HPA responses to stress (which is, of course, an inducible defense).

Maternal behavior in the rat permanently alters the development of hypothalamic-pituitary-adrenal responses to stress through tissue-specific effects on gene expression. The magnitude of the HPA response to stress is a function of the neuronal stimulation of hypothalamic corticotropin-releasing factor (CRF) release that then activates the pituitary-adrenal system, as well as modulatory influences, such as glucocorticoid negative feedback that inhibits CRF synthesis and release and thus dampens the HPA response to stress. The adult offspring of high-LG compared with low-LG mothers show increased hippocampal glucocorticoid receptor expression and enhanced glucocorticoid feedback sensitivity. Predictably, the offspring of high-LG mothers also show decreased hypothalamic CRF expression and more modest HPA responses to stress. Eliminating the difference in hippocampal glucocorticoid receptor levels abolishes the effects of early experience on HPA responses to stress in adulthood, suggesting that the difference in hippocampal glucocorticoid receptor expression serves as a mechanism for the effect of early experience on the development of individual differences in HPA responses to stress.

In vivo and in vitro studies suggest that maternal licking and grooming increases glucocorticoid receptor gene expression through increased hippocampal serotonin (5-HT) activity at 5-HT_7 receptors, and the subsequent intracellular enzyme activity. Both the in vitro effect of 5-HT, defined using primary hippocampal cell cultures, and the in vivo effect of maternal behavior on glucocorticoid receptor gene expression are accompanied by an increased hippocampal expression of the transcription factor, nerve growth factor–inducible factor A (NGFI-A). The noncoding (a segment of the DNA that does not code for a functional protein) exon 1 region of the hippocampal glucocorticoid receptor includes a promoter region, exon 1_7, containing a binding site for NGFI-A. Noncoding regions of the DNA do not code for functional proteins and are commonly contain sequences that regulate the expression of the "downstream" coding segment. The exon 1 region contains several promoter sequences that can alter gene expression. The exon 1_7 sequence functions as such a promoter, is apparently unique to neurons, and is more active in the offspring of high-LG mothers or following manipulations that increase maternal licking and grooming, which suggests that use of this promoter is enhanced as a function of maternal care. Moreover, maternal LG increases the binding of NGFI-A to the exon 1_7 sequence. Although these findings might explain the increased glucocorticoid receptor expression in the neonate, left unanswered is the question of how the effect of maternal care might persist into adulthood.

Transcription factors such as nerve growth factor–inducible factor A regulate gene expression, and thus provide a cellular interface between environment and gene. But the relationship is constrained. DNA operates within a chromatin context, which forms the DNA-packaging system inside the cell nucleus. Wrapped around the histone proteins, the DNA sequences that form our genetic code is only variably accessible to transcription factors. The positively charged histones and negatively charged DNA form bonds that preclude transcription factor binding to DNA sites. Enter the histone acetyl transferases (HATs) that acetylate (what else?) histone tails, neutralizing the charge, and relaxing the histone-DNA relationship to a state where transcription factors can enter the fray and bind to DNA sites. For those who considered DNA sites as mundane, passive recipients of intracellular influences, the science of chromatin remodeling through acetylation or other modifications renders the world a wonderfully interesting place.

Likewise, there are structural changes to DNA that result in far more stable silencing of DNA transcription. DNA methylation is a stable, epigenomic mark that occurs at cytosine nucleotides commonly found within promoter sequences. DNA methylation attracts a class of enzymes known as "histone deacetylases," which prevent histone acetylation, and preserve the tight histone-DNA relationship. DNA methylation is therefore associated with a stable suppression in gene transcription and is the pathway by which genes are turned off during early embryonic development. It may also be the mechanism by which maternal care during postnatal life can program the expression of specific genes in the brain and elsewhere.

In our studies, my colleagues and I focus on the methylation of the exon 1_7 glucocorticoid receptor promoter. The results reveal significant differences in the methylation of the exon 1_7 glucocorticoid receptor promoter sequence as a function of maternal care. Of greatest interest is the significant difference in a single cytosine within the NGFI-A consensus sequence (the DNA sequence to which NGFI-A binds), which is always methylated in the offspring of low-LG mothers, but rarely so in those of high-LG mothers. This difference in DNA methylation occurs at a single nucleotide and emerges over the first week of life, which corresponds perfectly to the time during which high-LG and low-LG mothers differ in maternal care. Moreover, an adoption study in which the biological offspring of high- or low-LG mothers were cross-fostered to either high- or low-LG mothers within 12 hours of birth produced a pattern of exon 1_7 glucocorticoid receptor promoter methylation that was associated with the rearing mother thus reversing the difference in methylation at the cytosine within the NGFI-A consensus sequence in animals born to low-LG, but reared by high-LG, mothers.

Such differences in cytosine methylation are functionally relevant. Both in vivo and in vitro studies have shown that the methylation of the critical cytosine within the NGFI-A consensus sequence eliminates binding of the transcription factor to the exon 1_7 sequence of the glucocorticoid receptor. Presumably, the offspring of the low-LG-ABN mothers thus lose the ability to increase hippocampal glucocorticoid receptor expression through NGFI-A activation.

The offspring of high-LG mothers exhibit increased hippocampal glucocorticoid receptor expression from the exon 1_7 promoter and dampened hypothalamic-pituitary-adrenal axis response to stress. The differential pattern of methylation of the exon 1_7 glucocorticoid receptor promoter is proposed as a critical mechanism. DNA methylation attracts histone deacetylases that stabilize the tight histone-DNA configuration and prevent transcription factors, such as NGFI-A, from binding to promoter sites. In support of this idea, we found that trichostatin A, a compound that inhibits histone deacetylases, reverses the differences in NGFI-A binding to the exon 1_7 promoter of the hippocampal glucocorticoid receptor gene in the offspring of low-LG-ABN mothers, increasing receptor expression and reversing the differences in HPA responses to stress. Thus DNA methylation does appear to be one mechanism for the enduring maternal effects on the development of defensive responses to threat in mammals.

Parenting as a Competitive Sport

Maternal effects on the expression of defensive responses, such as increased hypothalamic-pituitary-adrenal activity, are a common theme in biology. Alteration of the methylation status of targeted DNA sites in response to variations in environmental stimulation might ultimately be a process mediating such maternal effects. DNA methylation could serve as an intermediate process that imprints dynamic environmental experiences on the fixed genome resulting in stable alterations in phenotype.

But what are the origins of the individual differences in maternal behavior? Perhaps the pivotal feature of this model is the increased estrogen receptor expression in the medial preoptic area (mPOA) of the hypothalamus of high-LG mothers; the mPOA is heavily implicated in the expression of maternal behavior in the rat. The increased estrogen sensitivity enhances oxytocin activity in the mPOA that, in turn, increases dopamine release from the nucleus accumbens. The increased dopamine release in the nucleus accumbens then drives pup licking and grooming. Now all this is great fun if you enjoy the details of neuroendocrinology, which I do immensely. But I could easily forgive readers for wondering if we have not missed the essential question. Why are not all mothers equally investing in their offspring?

Anxious human mothers are generally less sensitive to their offspring. Lactating Bonnet monkeys that are chronically stressed postpartum develop far more contentious relationships with their infants (Coplan et al., 1996). Likewise, when my colleagues and I stressed normally high-LG-ABN dams postpartum, they became low-LG-ABN dams. For reasons that are very poorly understood at the level of mechanism, stress seems to consistently decrease parental investment in the young, resulting in patterns of parental care that increase stress reactivity in the offspring.

Environmental adversity is translated into a pattern of maternal care that enhances the defensive responses of the offspring and likely reflects a very adaptive pattern of development. Children inherit not only genes from their parents, but also an environment: Englishmen inherit England, as Francis Galton remarked. Under conditions of increased environmental demand, it is commonly in the animal's interest to enhance its behavioral responsivity (e.g., vigilance, fearfulness) as well as its endocrine (HPA and metabolic or cardiovascular) responsivity to stress. These responses promote detection of potential threat, avoidance learning, and metabolic or cardiovascular responses that are essential under the increased demands of the stressor. Because the offspring usually inhabit a niche that is similar to their parents, the transmission of these traits from parent to offspring could serve to be adaptive. The key issue here is that of the potential adaptive advantage of the increased level of stress reactivity apparent in the offspring of low-LG mothers. In the present context, the research of Farrington and colleagues

(1988) and Tremblay (e.g., Haapasalo & Tremblay, 1994) on young males growing up in impoverished, high-crime environments in urban environments provides an excellent illustration of the potential advantages of increased stress reactivity. In this environment, the shier and more timid males were most successful in avoiding the pitfalls associated with such "criminogenic" environments. Under such conditions a parental rearing style that favored the development of increased stress reactivity to threat would be adaptive. Thus it is understandable that parents occupying a highly demanding environment might transmit to their young an enhanced level of stress reactivity in "anticipation" of a high level of environmental adversity. Such a pessimistic developmental profile would be characterized by an increased corticotropin-releasing factor gene expression, and by patterns of gene expression that dampen the capacity of inhibitory systems, such as the hippocampal glucocorticoid receptor system. The quality of the environment influences the behavior of the parent, which in turn is the critical factor in determining whether development proceeds along an optimistic versus a pessimistic pattern of development. In mammals, as in the radish or water flea, parental signals serve as a "forecast" of the level of adversity that lies ahead. The obvious conclusion is that there is no single ideal form of parenting: various levels of environmental demand require different traits in the offspring. This is a simple, even obvious message, with significant social implications.

References

Agrawal, A. A., Laforsch, C., & Tollrian, R. (1999). Transgenerational induction of defences in animals and plants. *Nature, 401*, 60.

Champagne, F., Diorio, J., Sharma, S., & Meaney, M. J. (2001). Naturally occurring variations in maternal behavior in the rat are associated with differences in estrogen-inducible central oxytocin receptors. *Proceedings of the National Academy of Sciences, U.S.A., 98*, 12736–12741.

Coplan, J. D., Andrews, M. W., Rosenblum, L. A., Owens, M. J., Friedman, S., Gorman, J. M., et al. (1996). Persistent elevations of cerebrospinal fluid concentrations of corticotropin-releasing factor in adult nonhuman primates exposed to early-life stressors: implications for the pathophysiology of mood and anxiety disorders. *Proceedings of the National Academy of Sciences, U.S.A., 93*, 1619–1623.

Farrington, D. P., Gallagher, B., Morlly, L., St. Ledger, R. J., & West, D. J. (1988). Are there any successful men from criminogenic backgrounds? *Psychiatry, 51*, 116–130.

Francis, D. D., Diorio, J., Liu, D., & Meaney, M. J. (1999). Nongenomic transmission across generations in maternal behavior and stress responses in the rat. *Science, 286*, 1155–1158.

Haapasalo, J., & Tremblay, R. E. (1994). Physically aggressive boys from ages 6 to 12: Family background, parenting behavior, and prediction of delinquency. *Journal of Consulting and Clinical Psychology, 62*, 1044–1052.

Lewontin, R. C. (1980). Sociobiology: Another biological determinism. *International Journal of Health Services, 10*, 347–363.

Liu, D., Tannenbaum, B., Caldji, C., Francis, D., Freedman, A., Sharma, S., et al. (1997). Maternal care, hippocampal glucocorticoid receptor gene expression and hypothalamic-pituitary-adrenal responses to stress. *Science, 277*, 1659–1662.

2   Aggression, Serotonin, and Gene-Environment Interactions in Rhesus Monkeys

Stephen J. Suomi

Whether the features that differentiate us as individuals are largely determined by our genetic heritage (nature) or shaped by our personal experiences (nurture) has been debated at least since the time of Aristotle. Selective breeding was practiced by those who grew plants or raised animals long before anything was known about specific genes, and assertions by educators and philosophers alike that "the child is the father of the man" predated by centuries any formulation of explicit theories of reinforcement by twentieth-century behaviorists.

Although the nature-nurture debate is far from new, what *is* relatively new is an emerging realization among those who study development that the basic questions underlying the nature-nurture debate over the years may have been largely misguided. Instead of arguments as to whether behavioral and biological characteristics that appear during development are genetic in origin or the product of specific experiences, it is becoming increasingly apparent that *both* genetic *and* environmental factors play crucial roles in shaping individual developmental trajectories and that they may indeed actually *interact* in the process.

This essay traces a program of research that has focused on identifying certain genetic and environmental factors—and their possible interactions—that apparently predispose some rhesus monkeys to become excessively and inappropriately aggressive. The research was largely inspired by the late Dr. Markku Linnoila, who at the time of his death five years ago was the scientific director of the National Institute of Alcohol Abuse and Alcoholism (NIAAA) and was clearly expanding an already extraordinary research career. I first met Dr. Linnoila almost twenty years ago, when he was a recently appointed laboratory chief in the NIAAA and I was being recruited from the University of Wisconsin to develop a new laboratory in a different National Institute of Health, the National Institute of Child Health and Human Development (NICHD). Within minutes of being introduced to each other, we decided to form a long-term collaboration, wherein his laboratory would analyze cerebrospinal fluid concentrations of monoamine metabolites collected from rhesus monkeys to be reared in different physical and social environments at the new primate facility that was being developed in the Maryland countryside. Moreover, to promote and sustain our collaboration, he offered to provide postdoctoral support for my senior graduate student at Wisconsin, J. D. Higley. At that time, I had no idea how unusual this collaboration was, given the tradition of intense competition for resources between the different institutes within the National Institutes of Health (NIH). My collaborative efforts with Dr. Linnoila and with Dr. Higley, now a tenured scientist in the NIAAA, have actually expanded over the years; although Dr. Linnoila is no longer with us, his remarkable vision and spirit persist in full force.

The primate facility that was built in the Maryland countryside near the town of Poolesville enabled my colleagues and me to study monkeys growing up under conditions that simulate most basic aspects of their natural physical and social environments. In nature, rhesus monkeys reside in large social groups (troops), each comprising several different female-headed families (matrilines) across several generations of kin, plus numerous immigrant males. This pattern of social organization derives from the fact that rhesus monkey females stay in their natal troop for their entire lives whereas virtually all rhesus monkey males emigrate from their natal troop around the time of puberty, usually in their fourth or fifth year, and then join other troops. These troops are also characterized by multiple social dominance relationships, including distinctive hierarchies both between and within families, as well as a hierarchy among the immigrant adult males. Among those males, relative status seems to be largely a function of one's ability to join and maintain coalitions, especially with high-ranking females. In sum, the dominance status of any particular rhesus monkey within its troop depends not so much on how big and strong it is but rather who its family and friends are—and the latter is clearly dependent on the development of complex social skills during ontogeny.

Rhesus monkey infants spend virtually all of their first month of life in physical contact with their biological mother, during which time they form a strong and enduring specific attachment bond with her. In their second month of life, they begin exploring their immediate physical and social environment, using their mother as a "secure base" to support such exploration, and they also begin interacting with other troop members, especially peers. In subsequent months, play interactions with peers increase dramatically in both frequency and complexity and thereafter remain at high levels until puberty. Aggression first appears in a young monkey's behavioral repertoire around 6 months of age, typically in the context of rough-and-tumble play. The capability for aggression is crucial for survival in the wild, not only for defending oneself and offspring from predators and conspecific competitors but also in maintaining social order and enforcing the complex dominance hirearchies characteristic of all rhesus monkey troops. On the other hand, uncontrolled, unpredictable, and violent aggression within any troop could drive members apart and destroy it as a social unit. Therefore, aggression must be *socialized*—it must be minimized or at least largely ritualized in intragroup interactions but also must remain a viable response to counter external threats or other dangers. The socialization of aggression for young monkeys involves not only learning in which circumstances and toward which targets aggressive behavior might be appropriate, but also gauging the relative intensity of the attack or response called for and the appropriate time and means for terminating an aggressive bout or avoiding it altogether.

In 1986, Dr. Linnoila invited me to participate in a symposium reviewing current knowledge regarding a possible link between violent aggression exhibited by child, adolescent, and adult patients and deficits in their serotonergic functioning, as indexed by unusually low concentrations of the primary central serotonin metabolite 5-hydroxyindoleacetic acid (5-HIAA) in their cerebrospinal fluid (CSF). To prepare for the symposium, we collected and assayed CSF samples for 5-HIAA concentrations from a cross-sectional sample of infant, juvenile, and adult rhesus monkeys in our NICHD colony. We also had considerable background data regarding levels of aggression for each age-sex class within our monkey sample. Consistent with the extant human data, we found a striking *inverse* relationship between levels of intense physical aggression and 5-HIAA concentrations both within and between each age-sex class (Higley, Suomi, & Linnoila, 1990b). We also collected additional CSF samples from a subset of these subjects a year later in different social settings and found that individual differences in 5-HIAA concentrations were remarkably stable across both time and situation, suggesting that this measure of serotonergic functioning was traitlike in nature (Higley, Suomi, & Linnoila, 1990a).

In light of these findings, we explored this inverse relationship more fully in our rhesus monkey colony, essentially replicating and extending our initial cross-sectional findings in a series of prospective longitudinal studies. First, we found that individual 5-HIAA concentrations in the cerebrospinal fluid were remarkably stable from infancy to adolescence, such that values obtained as early as 14 days of age were significantly correlated with those obtained from the same subjects repeatedly up to 4 years of age. We also found that approximately 5–10 percent of our monkeys exhibited impulsive behavioral tendencies and general social incompetence. Both males and females in this subgroup became involved in a disproportionate number of aggressive exchanges with other group members and were less likely to engage in positive affiliative behaviors such as social grooming. These monkeys consistently had lower 5-HIAA concentrations in their cerebrospinal fluid than their peers of like age and gender (Higley & Suomi, 1996).

Many of the behavioral tendencies that distinguished impulsively aggressive monkeys from others in their social group appeared as early as 4 months of age and remained remarkably consistent throughout the whole of development. Young males who exhibited such patterns initially did so in the context of rough-and-tumble play with peers—their play tended to be excessively aggressive, often escalating inappropriately to actual aggressive exchanges. At later ages these same males were disproportionately likely to confront high-ranking adult males in their social group, often with physically damaging consequences for themselves (Higley & Suomi, 1996). Juvenile females with chronically low 5-HIAA concentrations in their cerebrospinal fluid were found to exhibit low levels of social grooming, and while they typically were involved in fewer overtly aggressive acts than their male counterparts, they tended to become relatively isolated socially as they were growing up, typically drifting to the bottom of the dominance hierarchy within their social group (Higley, King, et al., 1996).

Other longitudinal studies demonstrated that individuals with the lowest 5-HIAA concentrations in their cerebrospinal fluid were disproportionately likely to have poor state control and visual orienting capabilities during early infancy (Champoux, Suomi, & Schneider, 1994) and performed poorly on delay-of-gratification tasks during their juvenile years (Tsai, Bennett, Pierre, Shoaf, & Higley, 1999). In addition, they exhibited altered sleep patterns (Zajicek, Higley, Suomi, & Linnoila, 1997), as well as unusually high cerebral glucose metabolism under mild isoflourine anesthesia as adults (Doudet et al., 1995). These monkeys also tended to consume excessive amounts of alcohol when placed in a "happy hour" setting as adolescents and young adults (Higley, Hasert, Suomi, & Linnoila, 1991).

Given the apparent association of low 5-HIAA concentrations in the cerebrospinal fluid with a host of potentially problematic behavioral tendencies throughout development among monkeys maintained in captive environments, we wondered whether individuals with similar biobehavioral profiles could be found in wild populations of rhesus monkeys—and if so, what might the adaptive consequences be for such individuals?

Through Dr. Linnoila's good offices, we obtained access to a free-ranging population of approximately 4,000 rhesus monkeys who had been living for many years on an island off the South Carolina seacoast. These monkeys were provisioned but received no special veterinary treatment, and except for periodic trapping of specified individuals for biological sampling they were not subject to any experimental interventions. Analyses of CSF samples obtained from juvenile, adolescent, and adult male rhesus monkeys residing on this island revealed 5-HIAA concentrations closely resembling those obtained from males in our NICHD colony in terms of absolute values, age-related differences, and stability of individual differences across repeated sampling and across major developmental transitions.

Like their captive counterparts, those wild rhesus monkey juveniles with the lowest 5-HIAA concentrations frequently turned routine rough-and-tumble play bouts into episodes involving serious aggressive exchanges, and they also were more likely to commit obvious social blunders that typically elicited physical attacks from more socially dominant adults (Higley et al., 1992). Juvenile males with low 5-HIAA concentrations in their cerebrospinal fluid were also more likely to take long, potentially dangerous leaps from treetop to treetop, sometimes falling to the ground and injuring themselves (Mehlman et al., 1994). Ostracized by their peers and frequently attacked by adults of both genders, most of these young males were physically driven out of their natal troop prior to 3 years of age, long before the onset of puberty (Mehlman et al., 1995). These impulsive young males generally lacked the social skills to be able to join another troop, and most failed to survive to adulthood (Higley, Mehlman, et al., 1996).

How might specific genetic or environmental factors, or both, influence the development of excessive impulsive and aggressive behavioral tendencies and potential serotonergic dysfunction? Heritability analyses of our NICHD colony have demonstrated that individual differences in 5-HIAA concentrations are highly heritable among monkeys of similar age and comparable rearing background (Higley et al., 1993). On the other hand, both 5-HIAA concentrations and their above-described behavioral correlates are also clearly subject to major modification by early social experiences, particularly those involving attachment relationships. For example, rhesus monkeys raised from birth away from their biological mothers but in the continuous company of similarly reared age mates for their first 6 months of life typically develop behavioral and physiological patterns that seem to mimic those biobehavioral features characteristic of excessively aggressive monkeys observed in naturalistic settings (Suomi, 2000). Specifically, peer-reared monkeys consistently exhibit lower 5-HIAA concentrations in their cerebrospinal fluid than their mother-reared counterparts throughout development, as well as higher rates of impulsive aggression and excessive alcohol consumption in adolescence and early adulthood (Higley, Suomi, & Linnoila, 1996).

Clearly, *both* genetic and early experiential factors can influence whether a rhesus monkey will develop such biobehavioral characteristics. Do these factors operate independently, or do they interact in some fashion in shaping individual developmental trajectories? In the year before his untimely death, Dr. Linnoila helped us establish a collaboration with Dr. K. P. Lesch, a biological psychiatrist at the University of Würzburg, who was conducting both molecular and epidemiological studies focusing on the serotonin transporter gene (5-HTT). Considered a "candidate" gene for impaired serotonergic function, this particular gene has length variation in its promoter region that results in allelic variation in serotonin expression. A heterozygous "short" allele (LS) confers low transcriptional efficiency to the 5-HTT promoter relative to the homozygous "long" allele (LL), raising the possibility that low 5-HTT expression may result in decreased serotonergic function (Heils et al., 1996).

In collaboration with Dr. Lesch and his colleagues, my laboratory has recently demonstrated that the consequences of having the LS allele differ dramatically between peer-reared monkeys and their mother-reared counterparts. Peer-reared monkeys with the LS allele exhibit deficits in measures of neurobehavioral development during their initial weeks of life, reduced serotonin metabolism, and excessive aggression and alcohol consumption as adolescents compared with those possessing the LL allele. In contrast, mother-reared subjects with the LS allele are characterized by normal early neurobehavioral development, normal levels of aggression, and normal serotonin metabolism, as well as by a lower propensity for excessive alcohol consumption later in life than their mother-reared counterparts with the LL allele (Bennett et al., 2002; Champoux et al., 2002; Barr et al., in press).

One interpretation of these interactions between 5-HTT allelic status and early social rearing environment is that being reared by a competent mother appears to "buffer" potentially deleterious effects of the LS allele on serotonergic functioning and behavioral responsiveness. Indeed, it could be argued on the basis of these findings that, whereas having the "short" allele of the 5-HTT gene may well lead to psychopathology among monkeys with poor early rearing histories, it might actually be adaptive for monkeys who develop secure early attachment relationships with their mothers. The implications of these recent findings are significant with respect to the potential for cross-generational transmission of these biobehavioral characteristics, in that the attachment style of a monkey mother is typically "copied" by her daughters when they grow up and become mothers themselves (Suomi, 1999). If similar buffering is indeed experienced by the next generation of infants having the "short" allele of the 5-HTT gene (carrying the LS 5-HTT polymorphism), then having had their mothers develop a secure attachment relationship with their own mothers may well provide the basis for a nongenetic means of transmitting its apparently adaptive consequences to that new generation.

My colleagues and I are currently conducting parallel studies of other potential gene-environment interactions involving not only 5-HTT polymorphisms but also polymorphisms in other "candidate genes" such as MAO-A and the dopamine D1 receptor gene, and our findings to date suggest that such interactions are ubiquitous and can occur at a variety of points throughout development. We are also currently involved in collaborative studies investigating patterns of gene expression in different brain regions and how such patterns might be influenced by early experience. It is truly a shame that Dr. Linnoila is no longer around to assist us in these endeavors. I am certain that he would have been eager to press onward in the efforts he helped us begin back in 1986.

References

Barr, C. S., Newman, T. K., Becker, M. L., Parker, C. C., Champoux, M., Lesch, K. P., et al. (in press). Early experience and rh5-HTTPLR genotype interact to influence social behavior and aggression in nonhuman primates. *Genes, Brain, and Behavior.*

Bennett, A. J., Lesch, K. P., Heils, A., Long, J., Lorenz, J., Shoaf, S. E., et al. (2002). Early experience and serotonin transporter gene variation interact to influence primate CNS function. *Molecular Psychiatry, 17,* 118–122.

Champoux, M., Bennett, A. J., Lesch, K. P., Heils, A., Nielson, D. A., Higley, J. D., et al. (2002). Serotonin transporter gene polymorphism and neurobehavioral development in rhesus monkey neonates. *Molecular Psychiatry, 7,* 1058–1063.

Champoux, M., Suomi, S. J., & Schneider, M. L. (1994). Temperamental differences between captive Indian and Chinese-Indian hybrid rhesus macaque infants. *Laboratory Animal Science, 44,* 351–357.

Doudet, D., Hommer, D., Higley, J. D., Andreason, P. J., Moneman, R., Suomi, S. J., et al. (1995). Cerebral glucose metabolism, CSF 5-HIAA, and aggressive behavior in rhesus monkeys. *American Journal of Psychiatry, 152,* 1782–1787.

Heils, A., Teufel, A., Petri, S., Stober, G., Riederer, P., Bengel, B., et al. (1996). Allelic variation of human serotonin transporter gene expression. *Journal of Neurochemistry, 6,* 2621–2624.

Higley, J. D., Hasert, M. F., Suomi, S. J., & Linnoila, M. (1991). Nonhuman primate model of alcohol abuse: Effects of early experience, personality, and stress on alcohol consumption. *Proceedings of the National Academey of Sciences, U.S.A., 15,* 7261–7265.

Higley, J. D., King, S. T., Hasert, M. F., Champoux, M., Suomi, S. J., & Linnoila, M. (1996). Stability of individual differences in serotonin function and its relationship to severe aggression and competent social behavior in rhesus macaque females. *Neuropsychopharmacology, 14,* 67–76.

Higley, J. D., Mehlman, P. T., Taub, D. M., Higley, S., Fernald, B., Vickers, J. H., et al. (1996). Excessive mortality in young free-ranging male nonhuman primates with low CSF 5-HIAA concentrations. *Archives of General Psychiatry, 53*, 537–543.

Higley, J. D., Mehlman, P. T., Taub, D. M., Higley, S. B., Vickers, J. H., Suomi, S. J., et al. (1992). Cerebrospinal fluid monoamine and adrenal correlates of aggression in free-ranging rhesus monkeys. *Archives of General Psychiatry, 49*, 436–444.

Higley, J. D., & Suomi, S. J. (1996). Reactivity and social competence affect individual differences in reaction to severe stress in children: Investigations using nonhuman primates. In C. R. Pfeffer (Ed.), *Intense stress and mental disturbance in children* (pp. 3–58). Washington, DC: American Psychiatric Press.

Higley, J. D., Suomi, S. J., & Linnoila, M. (1990a). Parallels in aggression and serotonin: Consideration of development, rearing history, and sex differences. In H. van Praag, R. Plutchik, and A. Apter (Eds.), *Violence and suicidality* (pp. 245–256). New York: Bruner/Mazel.

Higley, J. D., Suomi, S. J., & Linnoila, M. (1990b). Developmental influences on the serotonergic system and timidity in the nonhuman primate. In E. M. Coccaro and D. L. Murphy (Eds.), *Serotonin in major psychiatric disorders* (pp. 27–46). Washington, DC: American Psychiatric Press.

Higley, J. D., Suomi, S. J., & Linnoila, M. (1996). A nonhuman primate model of Type II alcoholism? 2. Diminished social competence and excessive aggression correlates with low CSF 5-HIAA concentrations. *Alcoholism: Clinical and Experimental Research, 20*, 643–650.

Higley, J. D., Thompson, W. T., Champoux, M., Goldman, D., Hasert, M. F., Kraemer, G. W., et al. (1993). Paternal and maternal genetic and environmental contributions to CSF monoamine metabolites in rhesus monkeys (*Macaca mulatta*). *Archives of General Psychiatry, 50*, 615–623.

Mehlman, P. T., Higley, J. D., Faucher, I., Lilly, A. A., Taub, D. M., Vickers, et al. (1994). Low cerebrospinal fluid 5 hydroxyindoleacetic acid concentrations are correlated with severe aggression and reduced impulse control in free-ranging primates. *American Journal of Psychiatry, 151*, 1485–1491.

Mehlman, P. T., Higley, J. D., Faucher, I., Lilly, A. A., Taub, D. M., Vickers, J. H., et al. (1995). CSF 5-HIAA concentrations are correlated with sociality and the timing of emigration in free-ranging primates. *American Journal of Psychiatry, 152*, 901–913.

Suomi, S. J. (1999). Attachment in rhesus monkeys. In J. Cassidy & P. R. Shaver (Eds.), *Handbook of attachment: Theory, research, and clinical applications* (pp. 181–197). New York: Guilford Press.

Suomi, S. J. (2000). A biobehavioral perspective on developmental psychopathology: Excessive aggression and serotonergic dysfunction in monkeys. In A. J. Sameroff, M. Lewis, & S. Miller (Eds.), *Handbook of developmental psychopathology* (pp. 237–256). New York: Plenum Press.

Tsai, T., Bennett, A. J., Pierre, P. J., Shoaf, S. E., & Higley, J. D. (1999). Behavioral response to novel objects varies with CSF 5-HIAA concentrations in rhesus monkeys. *American Journal of Primatology, 49*, 109–110.

Zajicek, K., Higley, J. D., Suomi, S. J., & Linnoila, M. (1997). Rhesus macaques with high CSF 5-HIAA concentrations exhibit early sleep onset. *Psychiatric Research, 77*, 15–25.

3 A Balance Within: Dissecting Neural and Neuroendocrine Pathways That Transduce Signals from the Outside World

Esther M. Sternberg

The Two Cultures

In the mid-nineteenth century, the French physiologist Claude Bernard described the "milieu interne"—the balance of factors within the body that, together maintain a state of homeostasis when the organism is perturbed by outside destabilizing forces (Sternberg, 2001). How one moves from those outside forces that perturb the internal balance, and how one measures and defines mechanisms by which the body reestablishes equilibrium, are questions that philosophers, scientists, and physicians have grappled with for millennia prior to Claude Bernard and in the century and a half since. Scientists from opposite ends of the spectrum—the social sciences and the physiological and molecular sciences—often view these questions from their own particular perspectives and may not see the need to bridge the gap between disciplines, let alone ways to do so.

The Dilemma

In the social and behavioral sciences, external perturbations can be parsed into their individual components, observed, defined, and measured. In the physiological and molecular sciences, the complex interplay of molecules, hormones, neurotransmitters, and their receptors, as well as their interactions within and between cells, can all be studied to the minutest detail. But, unlike in nature, the two worlds do not often intermingle. Perhaps it is because it is difficult in a single experiment to move from the larger scale of the social world to the microscopic and submicroscopic scale of the cellular or molecular world. Perhaps it is because the time frame under which such external perturbations occur is so different from the time frames of the various bodily systems that have evolved to respond to them. Or perhaps it is because the outcome measures the two sets of disciplines grapple with are so different—abstract, intangible social interactions, as opposed to concrete, tangible chemicals and cells that can be isolated, weighed, and readily measured—the old Cartesian dilemma. Most likely, it is because we have not had sensitive-enough tools to address questions at both ends of the spectrum until quite recently. Whatever the reason, it is only lately that social scientists, neurobiologists, and immunologists have begun to tackle these questions collaboratively, using the most sensitive measures developed within each discipline.

From Immunology to Neuroendocrinology

My own research began from the perspective of immunologist, studying a focused animal model of inbred rat strains bred by immunologists for their relative susceptibility and resistance to autoimmune inflammatory disease. The notion that the endocrine system might play a physiological role in regulating the immune system did not occur to me until an unexpected event during a pharmacological experiment using these rat strains. It was in the course of testing the in vivo effects of an experimental serotonin antagonist that, in vitro, had blocked macrophage activation. To our great surprise, a strain usually resistant to developing inflammation, especially massive autoimmune inflammation—the Fischer rats—began dying rapidly in what appeared to be septic shock. It was all the more surprising because the serotonin antagonist had suppressed inflammation among immune cells in culture.

The Clues

To explain this mysterious outcome, my colleagues and I looked to the pharmacology of this drug in the nervous system, to the fact that it blocked the neuroendocrine (hypothalamic-pituitary-adrenal; HPA) stress response. That only the rats treated with both bacterial cell walls and serotonin antagonist died, and not those treated with either agent alone, told us that the drug, by itself, was not toxic, but was doing something to block response systems that ordinarily suppressed inflammation. These clues led us to hypothesize that the physiological difference between these two strains predisposing or protecting them from inflammation was related to their differential HPA-axis responsiveness (Sternberg, Hill et al., 1989; Sternberg, Young et al., 1989).

The Neuroendocrine Stress Response and Inflammatory Susceptibility

To test this hypothesis, we did a clinical endocrine workup of the hypothalamic-pituitary-adrenal axis in these rats. We found that, indeed, the animals resistant to autoimmune

inflammation had a hyperactive HPA axis, whereas the susceptible animals had an underactive one. Because of this, when
exposed to inflammatory stimuli such as bacterial cell walls, the
animals susceptible to autoimmune inflammation were unable
to make enough of the anti-inflammatory stress hormone
corticosterone, whereas the resistant animals made too much of
it, immediately shutting off inflammation as soon as it began.
By removing the anti-inflammatory effects of this stress hormone with drugs that prevented its release, we removed these
animals' main protective mechanism to shut off inflammation,
and they died in septic shock. We and others have gone on to
prove and re-prove this effect in many ways, turning animals
susceptible to autoimmune inflammation into ones resistant to
it by removing their adrenals or pituitaries or by using drugs
that block the effects of corticosterone (MacPhee, Antoni,
Mason, 1989; Sternberg, Hill et al., 1989; Edwards, Yunger,
Lorence, Dantzer, & Kelley, 1991; Ruzek, Pearce, Miller, & Biron,
1999; Gomez et al., 2003; for review, see Webster, Tonelli,
Sternberg, 2002).

An Animal Model to Study the Link between Biological Response Systems and Social Perturbations

The observation that the neuroendocrine stress response plays
a critical role in protecting animals from inflammation was the
first step in establishing an animal model that could be analyzed
at multiple levels to understand the many interactions between
external disturbing forces, such as social interactions, and internal correcting mechanisms, such as neuroendocrine and neural
response systems and immune responses. Thus it is possible in
a systematic and quantitative way to measure outcomes and

to intervene at multiple levels, including social, behavioral, physiological, neuroanatomical or neurochemical, neurohormonal, immune cellular and disease outcome (Sternberg, 1997; Sternberg & Gold, 2002; Webster et al., 2002). The ability to manipulate each of these interacting components systematically throughout development, under different hormonal and environmental conditions, allows us to evaluate the ways in which physiological and cellular response systems respond to physical, psychological, and social external perturbations in the environment.

From Genes to Environment

Such animal models also provide a method for systematically dissecting nature versus nurture questions in genetically homogeneous organisms where genetic contributions to defined traits can be identified. Numerous genetic linkage and segregation studies using multiple strains of rats, including our own in Lewis and Fischer rats, have shown that over 20 regions on 15 chromosomes contribute to inflammatory susceptibility and resistance (Remmers et al., 1996; Listwak et al., 1999). Mathematical analyses of such genetic data indicate that genetic factors contribute only to about 35 percent of the variance in expression of inflammatory disease. These complex illnesses are thus, multigenic and polygenic, with many genes, each having a small effect, contributing to final disease expression. This pattern of inheritance is characteristic of complex illnesses such as inflammatory arthritis, diabetes, cardiovascular disease, and hypertension. The low genetic contribution to expression of such diseases presents a challenge to genetic analyses aimed at identifying the gene or genes responsible for such traits. The corollary of this finding, that environmental factors must contribute to about 65 percent of the variance in expression of inflammatory disease, leads us to ask what those environmental factors might be.

By holding genetic variables constant, one can first define and then manipulate environmental factors that might contribute to variance in final disease expression. In my own research, the leap from focusing exclusively on the genetic and hormonal end of the spectrum to including the social interaction end occurred as a result of observations made during genetic linkage and segregation experiments. The first step in these experiments involves interbreeding two strains of rats or mice that each expressed the extremes of a given trait, in our case, high inflammation/low HPA axis and low inflammation/high HPA axis. Such intercrosses result in an "F1" generation—a generation whose inherited genes are derived in equal parts from mother and father of each parental strain. The F1 generation's genetic load therefore reflects equally the genes contributed by both parental strains and the quantitative trait expression should fall exactly halfway between both extremes. Any variance around the mean therefore reflects variance derived from so-called environmental variables, which are usually poorly defined.

To maximize chances of identifying candidate genes, geneticists generally try to minimize so-called environmental variability. On the other hand, sorting out which of the many potential environmental influences contribute to final disease susceptibility and outcome is at least as important, and potentially more useful from a disease intervention standpoint. Individual environmental variables for the disease trait can, at least potentially, be modified to reduce or prevent disease, whereas genes cannot. Among the environmental variables that could contribute to the sorts of variability we observed are in utero hormone exposures, stress in early development, and crowding or certain social interactions in adulthood.

From F1 Intercrosses to Maternal-Pup Interactions

The veterinarian assigned to perform the intercross studies in my laboratory, Maria Gomez, noticed that when she tried to wean the F1 pups from the mothers of the two different strains (high stress response/low inflammation versus low stress response/high inflammation), the mothers of the two strains behaved very differently. The mothers of one strain quickly hid their pups from Maria and prevented her from removing them, whereas the mothers of the other strain did not interfere with her at all. Under the supervision of Anthony Riley, an expert in animal behavior, Maria went on to systematically define the maternal behavior and maternal pup interactions in these strains. These studies revealed that the low–stress response/high-inflammation mothers (Lewis rats) exhibit efficient maternal behaviors, rapidly retrieving all pups scattered about the edge of the cage to quickly crouch and nurse. In contrast, the high–stress response/low-inflammation mothers (Fischer rats) completely ignore the pups for the entire 15-minute observation period (Gomez-Serrano, Sternberg, & Riley, 2002). Further cross-fostering studies revealed that genetic strain, maternal behavior, and gender factors contribute to final set point of the HPA-axis response in the adult animals, whereas cross-fostering has no effect on the inflammatory trait (Gomez-Serrano, Tonelli, Listwak, Sternberg, & Riley, 2001).

Broadening Approach to Research through Interdisciplinary Teams

Many factors influenced me in my journey from the narrowly focused thinking of cellular immunologist to thinking more broadly to incorporate principles of social neuroscience in the experimental paradigms that I study. One was the very first observation—so dramatic in its outcome—that drugs work differently in organisms than they do in isolated cells. This basic fact of biology, so obvious and yet so often ignored, tells us that we must develop methods for understanding the complex interplay of many biological factors at multiple levels, on the one hand, and individual molecular structures and genes, on the other. Although, to apply the best methodologies of each discipline to solve the problems at the interface of many, one must work in interdisciplinary teams, one cannot apply the principles of another discipline to one's own research without learning to identify which techniques of that discipline can be feasibly applied to the problems at hand. This requires becoming an "informed consumer" of many disciplines, while remaining an expert in one's own. There are many ways to achieve this—through seminars, workshops, or ongoing interdisciplinary collaborative groups. In my own experience, participation in a long-standing interdisciplinary collaborative group, the MacArthur Foundation's Mind Body Network (1995–2000), allowed me to interact with social neuroscientists, neurobiologists of emotions, animal etholo-gists, psychophysiologists, neuroimagers, endocrinologists, and psychiatric experts in sleep, hypnosis, and group therapy, greatly broadening my thinking both conceptually and technically.

The experience of learning the mind-set and experimental approach of another's discipline by grappling with scientific questions common to all is perhaps the most effective way of bringing the power of interdisciplinary teams to bear on complex multilevel questions. It is no longer possible, as it was in Claude Bernard's day and before, for one scientist to become expert in all disciplines required to solve a given problem. The wealth and depth of information, the distinctive language and technology in each discipline require that we each respect the other approaches and learn to work together to solve problems in a network where the whole is far greater than the sum of its parts. In the next century, many versions of such interdisciplinary scientific teams (see Zerhouni, 2003) will address the complex problems that result when different molecules within cells, different cell types, organ systems, individuals acting alone or in groups, and even whole populations interact simultaneously with each other and with factors in the environment. This approach will take the hard-to-grasp intangible phenomena of the social sciences, once characterized as "mysterious ethers," and connect them to the nerve pathways, cells, hormones, molecules, and receptors that transduce these signals from the outside environment to maintain a balance within.

References

Edwards, C. K., III, Yunger, L. M., Lorence, R. M., Dantzer, R., & Kelley, K. W. (1991). The pituitary gland is required for protection against lethal effects of *Salmonella typhimurium*. *Proceedings of the National Academy of Sciences, U.S.A., 88*, 2274–2277.

Gomez, S. A., Fernandez, G. C., Vanzulli, S., Dran, G., Rubel, C., Berki, T., et al. (2003). Endogenous glucocorticoids attenuate Shiga toxin-2-induced toxicity in a mouse model of haemolytic uraemic syndrome. *Clinical and Experimental Immunology, 131*(2), 217–224.

Gomez-Serrano, M., Tonelli, L., Listwak, S., Sternberg, E., & Riley, A. L. (2001). Effects of cross fostering on open-field behavior, acoustic startle, lipopolysaccharide-induced corticosterone release, and body weight in Lewis and Fischer rats. *Behavior Genetics, 31*(5), 427–436.

Gomez-Serrano, M. A., Sternberg, E. M., & Riley, A. L. (2002). Maternal behavior in F344/N and LEW/N rats. Effects on carrageenan-induced inflammatory reactivity and body weight. *Physiology and Behavior, 75*(4), 493–505.

Listwak, S., Barrientos, R. M., Koike, G., Ghosh, S., Gomez, M., Misiewicz, B., et al. (1999). Identification of a novel inflammation-protective locus in the Fischer rat. *Mammalian Genome, 10*(4), 362–365.

MacPhee, I. A. M., Antoni, F. A., & Mason, D. W. (1989). Spontaneous recovery of rats from experimental allergic encephalomyelitis is dependent on regulation of the immune system by endogenous adrenal corticosteroids. *Journal of Experimental Medicine, 169,* 431–445.

Remmers, E. F., Longman, R. E., Du, Y., O'Hare, A., Cannon, G. W., Griffiths, M. M., et al. (1996). A genome scan localizes five non-MHC loci controlling collagen-induced arthritis in rats. *Nature Genetics, 14*(1), 82–85.

Ruzek, M. C., Pearce, B. D., Miller, A. H., & Biron, C. A. (1999). Host defense: Endogenous glucocorticoids protect against cytokine-mediated lethality during viral infection. *Journal of Immunology, 162,* 3527–3533.

Sternberg, E. M. (1997). Emotions and disease: from balance of humors to balance of molecules. *Nature Medicine, 3*(3), 264–267.

Sternberg, E. M. (2001). *The balance within: The science connecting health and emotions.* New York: Freeman/Holt.

Sternberg, E. M., & Gold, P. W. (2002). The Mind-Body Interaction in Disease. *Scientific American, 12*(1), 82–89.

Sternberg, E. M., Hill, J. M., Chrousos, G. P., Kamilaris, T., Listwak, S. J., Gold, P. W., et al. (1989). Inflammatory mediator-induced hypothalamic-pituitary-adrenal axis activation is defective in streptococcal cell wall arthritis-susceptible Lewis rats. *Proceedings of the National Academy of Sciences, U.S.A., 86*(7), 2374–2378.

Sternberg, E. M., Young, W. S., III, Bernadini, R., Calogero, A. E., Chrousos, G. P., Gold, P. W., et al. (1989). A central nervous system defect in biosynthesis of corticotropin-releasing hormone is associated with susceptibility to streptococcal cell wall-induced arthritis in Lewis rats. *Proceedings of the National Academy of Sciences, U.S.A., 86*(12), 4771–4775.

Webster, J. I., Tonelli, L., & Sternberg, E. M. (2002). Neuroendocrine regulation of immunity. *Annual Review of Immunology, 20,* 125–163.

Zerhouni, E. (2003). Medicine: the NIH roadmap. *Science, 302*(5642), 63–72.

4 Protective and Damaging Effects of Stress Mediators

Bruce S. McEwen

The brain was once thought to have primarily descending influences on the body, and stressors of all varieties, to ignite a general and diffuse arousal reaction there. Based on our research and that of others, a very different picture of integrative physiology has emerged—the brain and body are in two-way communication via the autonomic nervous, endocrine, and immune systems; the social environment has a cumulative impact on physical and mental health and the progression of a number of specific diseases.

Selye's General Adaptation Syndrome in Relation to Allostasis

Hans Selye (1907–1983) is credited with introducing the concept of "stress" into popular as well as medical discussions. Before the enormous advances in biomedical research of the past five decades, which have added more detailed knowledge of the so-called stress hormones and their actions throughout the body, Selye (1936) used the emergency reaction of the sympathetic nervous system and adrenocortical system for his classic theory of stress. This has been captured in the classic "fight or flight" response of a gazelle chased by a lion. Selye postulated "the general adaptation syndrome," a stereotyped physiological response that takes the form of a series of three stages in the reaction to a stressor: (1) the *alarm reaction*, in which the adrenal medulla releases epinephrine, and the adrenal cortex produces glucocorticoids, promoting adaptation and restoring homeostasis; (2) *resistance*, in which defense and adaptation are sustained and optimal; (3) and, if the stress response persists, *exhaustion*, in which adaptive responding ceases, and illness, death, or both may follow.

How has this changed in light of new information? First, it is important to note that Selye's general adaptation syndrome is no longer interpreted to mean that there is a stereotyped response of stress mediators to all types of stress. Rather, there are different patterns of response of the hypothalamic-pituitary-adrenal (HPA) axis and the noradrenergic and adrenergic nerves that are related to the type of stressor (Chrousos, 1998; Goldstein, 1995). Another important qualification to the classic stress theory, is that "fight or flight" most accurately characterizes the response of male animals under threat, whereas the female response to non-life-threatening stress has been characterized by S. E. Taylor and colleagues (2000) as "tend-and-befriend, not fight-or-flight." Thus, although females do flee from extreme danger, gender differences need to be factored into the understanding of allostasis and allostatic load. These differences include not only the different perceptions and behavioral responses to stressors, as implied in the different terms, *tend and befriend* versus *fight or flight*, but also physiological differences in the regulation of mediators of allostasis. Estrogens appear to attenuate the HPA response to stress and preserve HPA regulation of cortisol release, in that postmenopausal women exhibit larger, age-related increases in cortisol secretion, higher 24-hour cortisol excretion, and a greater response to corticotropin-releasing hormone (CRH) stimulation than men of the same age (Van Cauter, Leproult, & Kupfer, 1996). Moreover, in response to the stress of a driving simulation challenge, postmenopausal women exhibited a greater HPA response than men (Seeman, Singer, & Charpentier, 1995). Furthermore, it has been shown that short-term estrogen replacement in postmenopausal women attenuates the glucocorticoid response to a psychological stress paradigm (Komersaroff, Esler, & Sudhir, 1999) and physical stress (Lindheim et al., 1992).

Finally, it is Selye's third stage, "exhaustion," that needs to be reinterpreted in light of newer knowledge that the stress mediators can have both protective and damaging effects depending on the time course of their secretion. Thus, rather than exhaustion of defense mechanisms, it is the stress mediators themselves that can turn against the body and cause problems.

Allostasis and Allostatic Load

In formulating ways of conceptualizing and measuring the underlying biological processes, my colleagues and I have introduced three concepts and terms, namely, *allostasis, allostatic load*, and *allostatic overload*, to allow for a more restricted and precise definition of the overused word *stress*, on the one hand, and to suggest how the essential protective and adaptive effects of physiological mediators that maintain homeostasis are, when mismanaged or overused, also involved in the cumulative wear and tear effects of daily life, on the other. By clarifying inherent ambiguities in the concept of homeostasis, these concepts and terms also clarify (and replace) aspects of Selye's "general adaptation syndrome."

Central to Seyle's integrative model of stress, the concept of homeostasis refers to the stability of physiological systems that maintain life, used here to apply strictly to a limited number of physiological variables (end points) such as pH, body temperature, glucose levels, and oxygen tension that are truly essential for life and are therefore maintained within narrow ranges around set points. These set points, and other boundaries of control, may themselves change with environmental conditions, however. Because the concept of homeostasis, as defined by Selye, does not explain these changes, we introduced another concept, allostasis, to refer to the superordinate system by which stability is achieved through change. There are primary mediators of allostasis such as, but not confined to, hormones of the hypothalamic-pituitary-adrenal axis, catecholamines, and cytokines. Allostasis also clarifies an inherent ambiguity in the concept of homeostasis by distinguishing between systems that are essential for life (*homeostasis*) and systems that keep those systems in balance (*allostasis*).

When set points or other boundaries of control vary beyond homeostatic mechanisms, these variables are referred to as "allostatic states." Originally proposed for understanding physiological aspects of drug abuse (Koob & LeMoal, 2001), an allostatic state results in an imbalance of the primary mediators reflecting excessive production of certain mediators and inadequate production of others. Examples are hypertension, a perturbed cortisol rhythm in major depression or after chronic sleep deprivation, chronic elevation of inflammatory cytokines and low cortisol in chronic fatigue syndrome, imbalance of cortisol, corticotropin-releasing hormone, and cytokines in the Lewis rat that increases risk for autoimmune and inflammatory disorders. Allostatic states can be sustained for limited periods provided that food intake or stored energy such as fat, or both, can fuel homeostatic mechanisms. If imbalance continues for longer periods and becomes independent of maintaining adequate energy reserves, then symptoms of allostatic overload appear. Abdominal obesity is an example of this condition. Allostatic states, therefore, refer to altered and sustained activity levels of the primary mediators, such as glucocorticosteroids, that integrate energetic and associated behaviors in response to changing environments, challenges such as social interactions, weather, disease, predators, and pollution.

Allostatic states can produce wear and tear on the regulatory systems of the brain and body. The terms *allostatic load* and *allostatic overload* refer to the cumulative result of an allostatic state. For example, fat stored by bears preparing for the winter, birds preparing to migrate, or fish preparing to spawn is allostatic load. It can be considered the result of the daily and seasonal routines organisms have to survive and to store extra energy needed for migrating, molting, breeding, and so on. Within limits, they are adaptive responses to seasonal and other demands. If, however, one superimposes on these additional loads of unpredictable events in the environment, disease, human disturbance, and social interactions, then allostatic load can increase dramatically and become allostatic overload, serving no useful purpose and predisposing the individual to disease.

What Are the Mediators of Allostasis?

Allostasis occurs in every cell and tissue of the body when it is exposed to a change in the external or internal environment. Most commonly, the mediators of allostasis include the stress

hormones, adrenalin and cortisol, and also the other components of both the sympathetic and the parasympathetic nervous
systems. Other mediators such as the hormones prolactin, oxytocin, and vasopressin are also secreted when the individual is
challenged. The immune system, which is innervated and influenced by virtually every hormone in the body, produces
cytokines and chemokines that influence many other tissues
and cells. Finally, the nervous system, source of the master
hormones that drive the endocrine system, also uses neurotransmitters and neuromodulators to communicate among
nerve cells and to respond to a changing environment. One of
the most important features of these mediators is that they
operate nonlinearly—that is, many of them influence each
other reciprocally.

Central Role of the Brain

The brain is both master controller of the nervous, endocrine,
and immune systems and a target of these systems, subject to
both protection and damage. Allostasis also applies not only to
circulating hormones but also to events that take place in organs
and tissues of the body. In the nervous system, neurotransmitters, released by neuronal activity, produce effects locally that
either propagate or inhibit further neural activity. Neurotransmitters and hormones are usually released during a discrete
period of activation and then are shut off. The mediators themselves are removed from the intracellular space by reuptake or
metabolism so as not to prolong their effects. When they are
not, however, there is allostatic overload and the brain is at
increased risk for damage (Lowy, Wittenberg, & Yamamoto,
1995).

Protection and Damage

Every system of the body responds to acute challenge with allostasis, putting out mediators that promote adaptation and survival. When these acute responses are overused or inefficiently managed, allostatic load results.

Thus the secretion of the stress hormones adrenalin and cortisol in response to an acutely threatening event promotes and improves memory for the situation so that the individual can stay out of trouble in the future, whereas, when the stress is repeated over many weeks, some neurons atrophy and memory is impaired, while other neurons grow and fear is enhanced (Roozendaal, 2000). Thus, too, acute stress promotes immune function by enhancing movement of immune cells to places in the body where they are needed to defend against a pathogen, whereas chronic stress suppresses immune function, using the same hormonal mediators (Dhabhar & McEwen, 1999).

For the cardiovascular system, we see a similar paradox. Getting out of bed in the morning requires an increase in blood pressure and a reapportioning of blood flow to the head so that we can stand up and not faint (Sterling & Eyer, 1988). Our blood pressure rises and falls during the day as physical and emotional demands change, providing adequate blood flow as needed. Yet repeatedly elevated blood pressure, particularly when combined with a supply of chemicals damaging to the coronary artery walls (cholesterol, lipids, oxygen-free radicals), promotes generation of atherosclerotic plaques (Manuck, Kaplan, Adams, & Clarkson, 1995). Beta adrenergic receptor blockers are known to inhibit this cascade of events and to slow down the atherosclerosis that is accelerated in dominant male cynomologus monkeys exposed to an unstable dominance hierarchy (Manuck, Kaplan, Muldoon, Adams, & Clarkson, 1991).

For metabolism, the paradox also is evident. Glucocorticoids, so named because of their ability to promote conversion of protein and lipids to usable carbohydrates, serve the body well in the short run by replenishing energy reserves after a period of activity, such as running away from a predator. By acting on the brain to increase appetite for food and to increase locomotor activity and food-seeking behavior (Leibowitz & Hoebel, 1997), glucocorticoids also regulate behaviors that control energy input and expenditure. Such regulation, however useful it may be when we do manual labor or play active sports, does not serve us well when we grab a pizza and a beer while watching television or writing a paper, particularly when these activities may also be generating psychological stress—for example, watching distressing news or worrying about getting the paper done in time. Inactivity and lack of energy expenditure creates a situation where chronically elevated glucocorticoids that may result from poor sleep, ongoing stress, or a rich diet can impede the action of insulin to promote glucose uptake. One of the results of this interaction is that insulin levels increase, and, when combined, elevated insulin and glucocorticoid levels promote both deposition of body fat and formation of atherosclerotic plaques in the coronary arteries (Brindley & Rolland, 1989). Whether psychological stress or sleep deprivation or a rich diet is increasing the levels of glucocorticoids, the consequences in terms of allostatic load are the same—insulin resistance and increased risk for cardiovascular disease. Thus catecholamines and the combination of glucocorticoids and insulin, though they perform important short-term adaptive roles, can have dangerous effects on the body over the long term and in combination with other chemicals (Brindley & Rolland, 1989).

Summary

In our new terminology, the first stage of Selye's general adaptation syndrome, the *alarm* reaction is reinterpreted as the process leading to adaptation, or *allostasis*, in which glucocorticoids and epinephrine, and other mediators, promote adaptation to the stressor. The second stage, of *resistance*, reflects the protective effects of the adaptation to the stressor. But if the alarm reaction is sustained and the levels of glucocorticoids and epinephrine are repeatedly elevated over many days, an allostatic state may ensue, leading to *allostatic load*, which replaces Selye's third stage, *exhaustion*, with the important distinction that this represents the almost inevitable wear and tear produced by repeated exposure to mediators of allostasis, that is, too much of a good thing. Thus Selye's diseases of adaptation are the result of the allostatic state leading to allostatic load and resulting in the exacerbation of pathophysiological change. Examples of allostatic load include the acceleration of athrosclerosis, abdominal obesity, and immunosuppression, as well as loss of minerals from bone, and atrophy or damage to the brain, especially the hippocampus (McEwen, 1998; Sapolsky, 1996).

References

Brindley, D., & Rolland, Y. (1989). Possible connections between stress, diabetes, obesity, hypertension and altered lipoprotein metabolism that may result in atherosclerosis. *Clinical Science, 77*, 453–461.

Chrousos, G. P. (1998). Stressors, stress, and neuroendocrine integration of the adaptive response. *Annals of the New York Academy of Sciences, 851,* 311–335.

Dhabhar, F., & McEwen, B. (1999). Enhancing versus suppressive effects of stress hormones on skin immune function. *Proceedings of the National Academy of Sciences,* U.S.A., *96,* 1059–1064.

Goldstein, D. S. (1995). *Stress, catecholamines, and cardiovascular disease.* New York: Oxford University Press.

Komesaroff, P. A., Esler, M. D., & Sudhir, K. (1999). Estrogen supplementation attenuates glucocorticoid and catecholamine responses to mental stress in perimenopausal women. *Journal of Clinical Endocrinology and Metabolism, 84,* 606–610.

Koob, G. F., & LeMoal, M. (2001). Drug addiction, dysregulation of reward, and allostasis. *Neuropsychopharmacology, 24,* 97–129.

Leibowitz, S. F., & Hoebel, B. G. (1997). Behavioral neuroscience of obesity. In G. A. Bray, C. Bouchard, and W. P. T. James (Eds.), *Handbook of obesity* (pp. 313–358). New York: Marcel Dekker.

Lindheim, S. R., Legro, R. S., Bernstein, L., Stanczyk, F. Z., Vijod, M. A., Presser, S., et al. (1992). Behavioral stress responses in premenopausal and postmenopausal women and the effects of estrogen. *American Journal of Obstetrics and Gynecology, 167,* 1831–1836.

Lowy, M. T., Wittenberg, L., & Yamamoto, B. K. (1995). Effect of acute stress on hippocampal glutamate levels and spectrin proteolysis in young and aged rats. *Journal of Neurochemistry, 65,* 268–274.

Manuck, S. B., Kaplan, J. R., Adams, M. R., & Clarkson, T. B. (1995). Studies of psychosocial influences on coronary artery atherosclerosis in cynomolgus monkeys. *Health Psychology, 7,* 113–124.

Manuck, S. B., Kaplan, J. R., Muldoon, M. F., Adams, M. R., & Clarkson, T. B. (1991). The behavioral exacerbation of atherosclerosis and its inhibition by propranolol. In P. M. McCabe, N. Schneiderman, T. M. Field, & J. S. Skyler (Eds.) *Stress, coping and disease* (pp. 51–72). Hove, England: Erlbaum.

McEwen, B. S. (1998). Protective and damaging effects of stress mediators. *New England Journal of Medicine, 338,* 171 179.

Roozendaal, B. (2000). Glucocorticoids and the regulation of memory consolidation. *Psychoneuroendocrinology, 25,* 213–238.

Sapolsky, R. M. (1996). Why stress is bad for your brain. *Science 273,* 749–750.

Seeman, T. E., Singer, B., & Charpentier, P. (1995). Gender differences in patterns of HPA axis response to challenge: MacArthur Studies of Successful Aging. *Psychoneuroendocrinology, 20,* 711–725.

Selye, H. (1936). A syndrome produced by diverse nocuous agents. *Nature 138,* 32.

Sterling, P., & Eyer, J. (1988). Allostasis: A new paradigm to explain arousal pathology. In S. Fisher, and J. Reason (Eds.). *Handbook of life stress, cognition and health.* (pp. 629–649). New York: Wiley.

Taylor, S. E., Cousino Klein, L. C., Lewis, B. P., Gruenewald, T. L., Gurung, R. A. R., & Updegraff, J. A. (2000). Biobehavioral responses to stress in females: Tend-and-befriend, not fight-or-flight. *Psychological Review, 107,* 411–429.

Van Cauter, E., Leproult, R., & Kupfer, D. J. (1996). Effects of gender and age on the levels and circadian rhythmicity of plasma cortisol. *Journal of Clinical Endocrinology and Metabolism, 81,* 2468–2473.

5   Oxytocin and the Prairie Vole: A Love Story

C. Sue Carter

Although, as a biologist by training, I did not set out to study love, more than a decade ago, I began to consider the possibility that my research did in fact have relevance for this concept. What first changed my thinking came in the mail, but, far from being a love letter, it was instead a negative review of a grant proposal I had submitted to the National Institutes of Health (NIH). The premise of this ill-fated proposal was that the hormone oxytocin could influence pair bond formation. The subjects for this research were socially monogamous rodents known as "prairie voles." My proposal did not mention love, nor, from my perspective at that time, did my research on voles have any but the most superficial bearing on the human concept of love. The media, however,—in particular, U.S.A. Today, which published an article on the morning of my grant review—had taken liberties with the prairie vole story, moving freely from rodent behavior into the realm of human emotion. Rather than discussing my proposal, the NIH review focused on the press coverage that had described oxytocin as the "hormone of love." My protests were futile. Over the intervening years, however, I came to accept the notion that, because the portions of neural systems necessary for love are ancient and shared by voles and humans, parallels between vole pair bonding and what humans call "love" might in fact exist.

But First, What Is Love?

Anyone who has fallen in love, held a newborn child, or lost a loved one has experienced the neurobiology of love. Definitions of love range from passion to compassion (Sternberg, 2000), and are beyond the scope of this essay. Although, from a biological perspective, love is a hypothetical construct and, as such, difficult to study, embedded in most definitions of human love is the concept of a social bond. Social bonds are also constructs, but these can be operationally defined by behavioral and physiological responses in the presence or absence of a loved one (for review, see Carter, 1998; Carter & Keverne, 2002; Carter, 2003). For example, the willingness to engage in selective social behaviors and the associated shifts in hormonal and neural activity may be relevant to the human experience of love.

Why Love and Be Loved

The origins of love and, more generally, sociality are most easily understood in the context of evolution. Mammalian reproduction demands, at a minimum, sexual behavior and the care of immature infants. Each of these requires sociality, and both are associated with selective social behaviors and attachments of varying temporal durations. Genetic investment in the form of direct or indirect parental investment has long been considered a driving force in the evolution of sociality. For many mammalian species, including our own, reproduction is most successful if there are two or more caretakers for the offspring.

Although the father is one obvious candidate for parental care, in the majority of mammalian species the involvement of the father in parenting is focused almost exclusively on accessing a mate and supplying sperm. On the other hand, in a small subset of animals, estimated at about 3–5 percent of mammalian species, that show the traits of social monogamy (Kleiman, 1977)—and which include, for example, marmosets and tamarins (New World primates), African wild dogs, certain species of rodents (such as prairie voles), and at least some humans—the father remains with his sexual partner after mating. His continued social involvement with the mother until the time of birth makes him available to be a caretaker for the young.

Social relationships and social bonds have benefits not only for the future of the species, but also in the here and now, improving individual survival. There is increasing evidence that social bonds protect and allow growth and restoration in the face of the stress of life and disease. For example, in humans a sense of social support is associated with a more successful recovery from cardiovascular disease, cancer, and mental illness and reduces the vulnerability to substance abuse. Epidemiological studies have repeatedly revealed that indices of social support are powerful predictors of vulnerability to many diseases (for review, see Uchino, Cacioppo, & Kiecolt-Glaser, 1996; Ryff & Singer, 1998). Although these studies leave little doubt that social bonds provide emotional and physical health benefits, they do not supply the mechanisms for such effects.

The benefits of sociality and social support may be of particular importance in mammals. In fact, the taxonomy of Mammalia is based on the nutritional support that passes in the form of milk from the mammalian mother to her immature infant. Among mammals, including humans, this support extends to selective sociality and caretaking indicative of social bonds. In a restricted number of species, including prairie voles, selective and enduring social relationships also are present between adults. Around these relationships families can emerge, consisting of the parents and their offspring, as well as other related or unrelated individuals (Carter & Getz, 1993).

Social bonds are interwoven with the capacity to adapt to an ever changing and challenging environment. Through the study of social bonds and the mechanisms that lead to the formation of such bonds, we can come to understand the physiological processes that allow humans to feel love, to express love, and to benefit physically and emotionally from both giving and receiving love.

How Do Social Bonds Protect?

To answer this question with the tools of science, it is necessary to understand that, like disease, love and social bonds are based on physiological processes that are regulated and experienced by the central and autonomic nervous system. Although it can certainly be argued that human consciousness is necessary to understand the concept of love, because human and nonhuman mammals share positive social interactions and social bonds, we can use knowledge of the natural history of social bonds among other mammals to predict the conditions and neuroendocrine mechanisms that will facilitate or block social engagement and the formation of social bonds among all mammals.

In mammals, new social attachments are more likely to be formed during or after periods of vulnerability, including birth, lactation and nursing, and sexual interactions, and especially after periods of stress or distress. The mother-child interaction, following the stress of birth and perhaps reinforced by nursing, is powerful evidence both that love exists and that it can be influenced by the biological events surrounding birth. Novelty or stress can help humans to form social bonds, a fact that is incorporated in the courtship traditions of many cultures. The combined effects of intense experiences followed by a physiological sense of safety seem to be present in many situations that lead to social bond formation.

Oxytocin—A Hormone of Love?

One uniquely mammalian hormone, oxytocin, is associated with lactation and birth, as well as the modulation of reactions to stress. Oxytocin is made in and acts on the brain, especially in the hypothalamus and areas of the nervous system that influence emotions. Oxytocin also has been implicated in various forms of positive social interactions including social bonding. Remarkably, this same hormone has the capacity to produce behavioral and physiological calming (Uvnas-Moberg, 1998).

The following features of the actions of oxytocin—derived primarily from animal research—suggest a role for oxytocin in social bonds and social support (for review, see Carter, 1998). Treatment with oxytocin quickly facilitates positive social behaviors, including selective partner preferences (Williams, Insel, Harbaugh, & Carter, 1994) and maternal behavior (Pedersen, 1997; Carter & Keverne, 2002). Chronic exposure to oxytocin is capable of down-regulating or buffering the response to stressors and the reactivity of the autonomic nervous system, including heart rate and blood pressure (Uvnas-Moberg, 1998). Oxytocin is released during positive social interactions and may permit social interactions without fear (Porges, 2001). Growth and restoration are facilitated by oxytocin. In rats, touch and massage (presumably in a context of perceived safety) can release oxytocin, which in turn may feed back to the nervous system to further enhance relaxation (Uvnas-Moberg, 1998). Of particular relevance to the integrative effects of oxytocin is the fact that this hormone has only one known type of receptor. Thus oxytocin is an excellent candidate for the integration of emotional experiences with the physiological processes through which love bestows its benefits.

Is Oxytocin *the* Love Hormone?

The unique actions of oxytocin seem to qualify this peptide as a central element in the neurobiology of attachment. However, many hormones and neural systems are involved in what we humans call "love." For example, the chemistry of reward is integral to the processes that allow attachments to form. Central to theories of reward is the catecholamine dopamine. In prairie voles, dopamine-oxytocin interactions have been implicated in the formation of social bonds in both sexes (Wang et al., 1999; Aragona, Liu, Curtis, Stephan, & Wang, 2003). Not all species of mammals have an anatomical association between dopamine and oxytocin; the colocalization—or alternatively, lack of colo-calization—of these chemicals may account in part for species differences in the capacity to form social bonds. Consistent with such differences, receptors for oxytocin and dopamine in rats and nonmonogamous voles are not colocalized in classic reward pathways (Insel, 2003). Conversely, the chemistry of love shares common elements with addiction (such as reliance on dopamine), which may ultimately help us to understand the causes of substance abuse. For example, disruption or the absence of social bonds is associated with anxiety and vulnerability to substance abuse, and the most effective treatments for addiction often incorporate social support.

On the other hand, many of the effects of oxytocin are most readily apparent following anxiety or stress, such as the events associated with birth. The hormones typically associated with stressful experiences include corticotropin-releasing hormone (CRH; a hypothalamic peptide capable of regulating the pituitary and adrenal glands) and adrenal steroids, including the glucocorticoids (specifically, corticosterone or cortisol). Glucocorticoids are released in response to various stressors and, conversely, may affect reactions to stress. In addition, catecholamines, including dopamine and the related hormone norepinephrine, are typically associated with increased mobilization and with the regulation of reward. The compounds are made both in the brain and adrenal gland and may play a role in the release of oxytocin. In addition, the binding of oxytocin to its receptor is increased by the presence of glucocorticoids, especially in the amygdala (Liberzon and Young, 1997). Perhaps anxiety or fear sets the stage for love, and oxytocin, released following exposure to stress hormones, helps to reduce anxiety or fear, especially in pair-bonding species. At the same time, the rewarding effects of dopamine could serve to cement relationships and enhance emotional feelings associated with love.

Are There Sex Differences in the Mechanisms of Love?

In male prairie voles, stressful experiences as well as adrenal steroids and the corticotropin-releasing hormone can facilitate pair-bonding (A. C. DeVries, M. B. DeVries, Taymans, & Carter, 1996; A. C. DeVries, Guptaa, Cardillo, Cho, & Carter, 2002). In female prairie voles, comparable stressful experiences or treatment with adrenal hormones inhibited female-male pair-bonding. Oxytocin's release also may be inhibited by stress.

In contrast, the related peptide vasopressin may be released during periods of self-defense and stress. The physiological actions of vasopressin (including increased heart rate, blood pressure, and water retention) may permit mobilization and self-defense. Although it is structurally similar to oxytocin (differing by only two amino acids), many of the physiological effects of vasopressin are opposite to those of oxytocin. Moreover—and of potential importance to understanding sex differences in love—vasopressin is androgen dependent and more abundant in males. Brain areas, including the amgydala, in which vasopressin is synthesized, are anatomically associated with functions, such as defensive vigilance, that may be more likely in males than females. Both oxytocin and vasopressin can influence social bonds in both sexes (Cho, A. C. DeVries, Williams, & Carter, 1999), although males—with more androgen and more endogenous vasopressin—may be more reliant than females on the latter peptide (Winslow, Hastings, Carter, Harbaugh, & Insel, 1993; Williams et al., 1994). The current data, drawn from animals, support the hypothesis that males remain capable of forming heterosexual social bonds under conditions of mobilization and arousal—possibly implicating vasopressin as well as other stress hormones. In contrast, the conditions that lead to enduring social bonding in females may require neural states associated with immobilization without fear (Porges, 2001). It is under these conditions that oxytocin may be especially critical.

Is There a Neurobiology of Love?

Simply stated, yes. Even though the experience of love and the causes and effects of social bonds are based on ancient neural and endocrine systems, however, the exact chemistry of human love remains to be described. Research on this topic is in its infancy and is limited by methodology and ethical considerations. Most of what is known comes from either correlational studies of changes in blood or brain activity, or is based on inferences from animal models. This research suggests that oxytocin and related hormones play a central role in the neurobiology of love, providing an intriguing link to mechanisms through which social bonds and social support may be physically and emotionally protective.

Acknowledgments

This essay is dedicated to Stephen Porges, who inspired my understanding of love as an emotional and physiological haven from the stress of life. I also wish to express gratitude to my colleagues and students, who provided many insights and the hard work necessary to test hypotheses regarding the neurobiology of love and social support, and to the National Institute of Mental Health, the National Institute of Child Health and Human Development, the National Alliance for Autism Research, and the Institute for Research on Unlimited Love, whose grants made this work possible.

References

Aragona, B. J., Liu, Y., Curtis, J. T., Stephan, F. K., & Wang Z. (2003). A critical role for nucleus accumbens dopamine in partner-preference formation in male prairie voles. *Journal of Neuroscience 23*, 3483–3490.

Carter, C. S. (1998). Neuroendocrine perspectives on social attachment and love. *Psychoneuroendocrinology, 23,* 779–818.

Carter, C. S. (2003). Developmental consequences of oxytocin. *Physiology and Behavior. 79,* 383–397.

Carter, C. S., & Getz, L. L. (1993). Monogamy and the prairie vole. *Scientific American, 268(6),* 100–106.

Carter, C. S., & Keverne, E. B. (2002). The neurobiology of social affiliation and pair bonding. In D. Pfaff et al. (Eds.) *Hormones, brain and behavior* (Vol. 1, pp. 299–337). San Diego: Academic Press.

Cho, M. M., DeVries, A. C., Williams, J. R., & Carter, C. S. (1999). The effects of oxytocin and vasopressin on partner preferences in male and female prairie voles (*Microtus ochrogaster*). *Behavioral Neurosciences, 113,* 1071–1080.

DeVries, A. C., DeVries, M. B., Taymans, S. E., & Carter, C. S. (1996). Stress has sexually dimorphic effects on pair bonding in prairie voles. *Proceedings of the National Academy of Sciences, U.S.A., 93,* 11980–11984.

DeVries, A. C., Guptaa, T., Cardillo, S., Cho, M., & Carter, C. S. (2002). Corticotropin-releasing factor induced social preferences in male prairie voles. *Psychoneuroendocrinology, 27,* 705–714.

Insel, T. R. (2003). Is social attachment an addictive process? *Physiology and Behavior, 79,* 351–357.

Kleiman, D. (1977). Monogamy in mammals. *Quarterly Review of Biology, 52,* 39–69.

Liberzon, I., & Young, E. A. (1997). Effects of stress and glucocorticoids on CNS oxytocin receptor binding. *Psychoneuroendocrinology, 22,* 411–422.

Pedersen, C. A. (1997). Oxytocin control of maternal behavior: Regulation by sex steroids and offspring stimuli. *Annals of the New York Academy of Sciences, 807,* 126–145.

Porges, S. W. (2001). The polyvagal theory: Phylogenetic substrates of a social nervous system. International *Journal of Psychophysiology*, *42*, 123–146.

Ryff, C. D., & Singer, B. (1998). The concept of positive human health. *Psychological Inquiries 9*, 1–19.

Sternberg, R. J. (2000). *Cupid's arrow: The course of love through time*. New York: Cambridge University Press.

Uchino, B. N., Cacioppo, J. T., & Kiecolt-Glaser, J. K. (1996). The relationship between social support and physiological processes: A review with emphasis on underlying mechanisms and implications for health. *Psychological Bulletin*, *119*, 488–531.

Uvnas-Moberg, K. (1998). Oxytocin may mediate the benefits of positive social interaction and emotions. *Psychoneuroendocrinology*, *23*, 819–835.

Wang, Z., Yu, G., Cascio, C., Liu, Y., Gingrich, B., & Insel, T. R. (1999). Dopamine D2 receptor-mediated regulation of partner preferences in female prairie voles (*Microtus ochrogaster*): A mechanism for pair bonding? *Behavioral neuroscience*, *113*, 602–611.

Williams, J. R., Insel, T. R., Harbaugh, C. R., & Carter, C. S. (1994). Oxytocin administered centrally facilitates formation of a partner preference in female prairie voles. *Journal of Neuroendocrinology*, *6*, 247–250.

Winslow, J. T., Hastings, N, Carter, C. S., Harbaugh, C. R., & Insel, T. R. (1993). Central vasopressin mediates pair bonding in the monogamous prairie vole. *Nature*, *365*, 545–548.

6 On Pheromones, Vasanas, Social Odors, and the Unconscious

Martha K. McClintock

Social regulation of biology is fundamental to social neuroscience, providing an essential counterbalance to traditional approaches that focus on biological mechanisms of social behavior. Chemical signals exchanged among members of a social group, termed *social chemosignals*, are a route by which social interactions and information can regulate both neural and endocrine events. Of particular interest are pheromones and vasanas, social chemosignals operating without conscious detection to regulate the nervous and endocrine systems as well as emotional reactions to social encounters.

Ovarian Primer Pheromones

Social chemosignals that regulate specific neural and hormonal mechanisms underlying fertility, behavior, and development are termed *pheromones*. When ovarian follicles are ripening, women produce pheromones that accelerate ovulation in other women and shorten their menstrual cycles (McClintock, 2002). In contrast, when women ovulate, their pheromones have the opposite effect on other women, delaying ovulation and lengthening menstrual cycles.

Levels of Organization

An ovarian pheromone is described most simply in the artificial context of a unidirectional dyad—a pheromone donor and receiver. But because the phenomenon of ovarian pheromones includes bidirectional interactions, it must be described at the social level of organization. In groups, the effect of pheromones becomes more varied and complex. For example, when women spend time together, their menstrual cycles are more likely to synchronize than those of a random sample of women in the same population (A. Weller & L. Weller, 2002; L. Weller, A. Weller, Koresh-Kamin, & Ben-Shoshan, 1999). But this is not always the case (McClintock, 1998).

Research with a rat model and computer simulations reveals two possible reasons for this apparent inconsistency. First, as in other coupled oscillator systems that exchange phase advance and delay signals, the group can synchronize, particularly when there are few individual differences in the strength of interactions. But when the interactions between some members are stronger than others, then synchrony is not only weaker, but cycles of the group can become asynchronous, or even stabilize without changing their initial relationship. Second, these different outcomes at the social level are predicted by the initial phase relationships of the group's ovarian cycles when they begin to interact. For example, if groups are partially asynchronous to start with, they become asynchronous.

Causes

In ovarian pheromonal communication, causation is downward from social to biological levels of organization, rather than upward. Social interactions are the mechanisms that change the ovary; women do not choose their friends based on the timing of their menstrual cycles. The cascade of mechanism begins at the social level of organization, mediated by pheromones changing the pulsatile release of luteinizing hormone (LH; Shinohara, Morofushi, & Kimura, 1999) and regulating ovulation (Stern & McClintock, 1998). Indeed, it is the social pattern of ovarian cycles that determines the resultant level of synchrony.

What is the function of ovarian pheromones? Do they have consequences that enhance survival or number of grandchildren, and thereby increase this trait in the population? The answer rests on recognizing that the ovarian cycle is a modern biological luxury, enabled by good nutrition, lack of physical and social stressors, and contraception (McClintock, 1998). Indeed, in traditional societies where food resources are scarce, fertility is highly seasonal and women may go more than a year without menstruating if crops fail. It has been estimated that, within the past 200 years, women have changed from having regular menstrual cycles for a total of three years to having them for more than 35 years. Thus the regulatory mechanisms for ovulation likely evolved in the context of a birth cycle: conception, pregnancy, and lactation. After puberty, ovulation would occur only after an infant was weaned and then only when women had sufficient food to regain body fat.

An animal model provides valuable clues to the function of pheromones (McClintock, 2000). Female rats conceiving and delivering pups within two weeks of each other rear their offspring communally, taking turns nursing. At weaning, these pups weigh more than those raised by a singleton mother, who expends more effort nursing. In stark contrast, two-thirds of the litters born asynchronously—far apart in time—are lost to predation. These pups are more likely to be females and are small at weaning. The function of ovarian pheromones then may have been selected in the context of coordinating birth cycles with the social world.

Indeed, birth and ovarian cycles have many neuroendocrine mechanisms in common. Pregnant rats produce pheromones that enhance ovulation in other rats. But once they are lactating, their pheromones disrupt and lengthen the cycles of other females. Compounds from breast-feeding women have similar disruptive effects, increasing variance in cycle length threefold.

Time Spans

Ovarian pheromones do not just operate in young adulthood. Indeed, as discussed above, their mechanisms and functions may be revealed more clearly in time spans other than the momentary time frame of minutes, hours, or days during adulthood. These same pheromonal mechanisms regulate the length of the reproductive life span, which is a powerful determinant of lifetime fitness in many mammals. Living in groups during puberty regularizes cycles disrupted by prenatal exposure to androgens (Zehr, Gans, & McClintock, 2001). Socially isolated animals, living without pheromonal and other social signals in middle age, suffer accelerated reproductive senescence.

Finally, it is the evolutionary time frame in which the function of these pheromones is played out. In constructing testable hypotheses, there is enormous power in recognizing how the same social, pheromonal, and neuroendocrine mechanisms are manifest in different contexts, and that selection may operate in only a subset. For example, ovarian pheromones may have evolved in humans to regulate puberty, ensuring that girls incur the considerable risks of reproduction in a supportive social and physical environment. As in other mammals, lactating human mothers could suppress the fertility of their daughters, ensuring that they help care for their siblings (McClintock, 2000). Changing the time of ovulation by a few days in women with spontaneous menstrual cycles may be as epiphenomenal as the menstrual cycle itself (McClintock, 1998).

Perspectives

Although the preovulatory surge of luteinizing hormone is measured from the objective (i.e., third-person) perspective, as is the social network within which pheromones are exchanged, the perception of these chemosignals can only be assessed from a subjective (i.e., first-person) perspective, raising the interesting question of what role conscious perception plays in the action of pheromones. Animal pheromones do not rely on odor. Indeed, in marked contrast to odors, one cannot condition responses to a pheromone or show stimulus generalization

Women do not identify ovarian pheromones as human odors (Stern & McClintock, 1998). Moreover, when women are exposed to compounds from breast-feeding women, they fail to detect any odor at all half of the time, just as they do when exposed to the control solution of potassium phosphate. And when they do detect an odor, they are as likely to say it is associated with something else as with humans. Moreover, women's endocrine response is independent of their ability to detect an odor (Jacob et al., 2003). Thus the effects of social interactions on neuroendocrine function are mediated by pheromones without conscious awareness by the group members.

Vasanas: Social Interactions and Moods

Social chemosignals can also modulate emotional responses to social interactions without being consciously detected as odors.

Androstadienone is a natural steroid secreted in human sweat, saliva, urine, and semen. Less than 9 nanomoles, the amount in a tenth of a drop of sweat, is sufficient to modulate emotional reactions to being in a laboratory experiment, preventing the degradation in mood that occurs over hours of filling out forms and reading bland material (McClintock, 2000). It also modulates sympathetic tone, release of cortisol, and glucose utilization in specific, yet widely distributed areas of the brain (Jacob, Kinnunen, Metz, Cooper, & McClintock, 2001). Yet the steroid cannot be detected as an odor in these small amounts, although it does have an odor at higher concentrations. Nonetheless, it is not at all clear whether this steroid is a behavioral pheromone, as some entrepreneurial fragrance companies claim, or a new type of social chemosignal (Jacob, Zelano, Hayreh, & McClintock, 2002). The four dimensions used above to discuss pheromones (levels of organization, causes, time spans, perspectives; Goldin-Meadow, McClintock, & Wimsatt, 2004) are a powerful tool for disentangling the essential questions in this newly emerging area of social neuroscience.

Levels of Organization

As with pheromones, at least four levels of organization are involved: social interactions, individual psychological responses, hormonal and neural events, and molecular biology. With the social chemosignal androstadienone, the social level of organization is involved not only because social groups share molecules, but also because social context modulates responses. When a man runs the experiment, women experience a change in both mood and sympathetic tone. But when women are tested by another woman, neither response is detected (Jacob et al., 2001).

This is a classic question for social psychologists. What about the social interaction with a man creates a psychological state that is modulated by androstadienone? Is it his personal characteristics or his gender? Or is the most parsimonious explanation at the level of the individual's psychological state, which could occur even when a woman is alone? Alternatively, is responding to androstadienone the "default," and do social interactions with another woman preclude the response?

Causes

As with pheromones, the mechanisms, that is, the antecedent events that cause the phenomenon (Goldin-Meadow et al., 2003), involve downward causation from the social level of shared social chemosignals to the changes in mood and underlying neural and endocrine events. The chemosignal is androstadienone, which is effective even through passive inhalation, when a saturated swab is waved under the nose—direct application is not necessary.

Understanding the mechanism is a further clue to the nature of this social chemosignal. Most behavioral pheromones in mammals act via the limbic system, particularly the hypothalamus, to increase social contact, sexual behavior, aggression, or fear (McClintock, 2002). Given that androstadienone modulates mood and does not release a fixed action pattern or a specific social cognition, we hypothesized that the prefrontal cortex would mediate the response (see Davidson, essay 7, this volume). On the other hand, the action of the social chemosignal modulated the reaction to participating in an experiment, leading my colleagues and me to also hypothesize that androstadienone modulates multiple aspects of the cortex engaged with the particular task at the focus of attention.

Positron-emission tomography measuring glucose utilization during the first 20 minutes of androstadienone exposure supported all three hypotheses (Jacob et al., 2001). While women were sitting still in front of a computer screen working on a visual discrimination task by moving a mouse, androstadienone changed glucose utilization in widespread areas of the brain specific to this visuomotor task. Changes in the visual cortex, the parietal cortex, thalamus, basal ganglia, premotor cortex, and cerebellum are all involved in the visuomotor task. In addition, changes in the prefrontal cortex, cingulate, hypothalamus, and amygdala are consistent with emotional regulation.

Identifying these neural mechanisms informs hypotheses about the function of this social chemosignal. It is not likely limited to heterosexual encounters, as others assume (Jacob, Zelano, Hayreh, & McClintock, 2002). Indeed, in men, the same compound decreases mood and increases sympathetic activity. Rather, it may serve to modulate emotional responses in a wide variety of social encounters. In particular, its function may be to allocate attention and cognitive resources, particularly when tasks are emotional, or are being done by an emotionally interconnected social group.

Time Spans

The momentary time span is used to distinguish primer and releaser pheromones. Endocrine primer pheromones typically work over several minutes, hours, and days. Behavioral releaser pheromones, however, can work within seconds to release action patterns, such as a male moth flying upwind to find the female releasing her sex attractant. Androstadienone modulates emotional responses, which are detectable within ten minutes and lasting up to 9 hours with a single exposure. It also prevents the drop in cortisol normally seen when a person sits down and relaxes, and subtly changes sympathetic tone, detectable while reading. Therefore, if androstadienone is a pheromone, its time frame of action does not fall into either of the classic types.

Thinking about androstadienone's function, operating across generations in evolutionary time, we are both informed and constrained by understanding its mechanisms. The modulation of brain areas involved in visuomotor tasks suggests that evolutionary fitness of this compound should be framed, not only narrowly in terms of sexual selection and mating, but also more broadly in its effects on the efficacy of a social group undertaking complex and demanding tasks. Thus it may have its primary function in childhood or in mediating the effects of social embeddedness on health and aging, and may not have been selected only in the context of young adults (see Berntson and Cacioppo, essay 9, this volume).

Perspectives

From the objective perspective, androstadienone has been chemically identified and purified and thus can be presented in precisely known amounts. At high concentrations, from the subjective perspective, it is consciously perceived as an odor, smelling musky and sweet to some, and slightly urinous to others, and it is often associated with the odor of men. But in nanomolar amounts, well below the threshold of detection and heavily masked with clove oil, it nonetheless affects people's mood and, more impressively, glucose utilization throughout the brain even when they cannot report a change in mood.

Clearly, androstadienone is an unconscious social chemosignal. But to describe its as having an "unconscious" or "subthreshold" odor is a contradiction in terms, because odors are by definition percepts caused by a chemical compound. On the other hand, its functions and mechanisms are not exactly like those of classic pheromones, nor do we yet have evidence that it modulates behavior in contexts in which it would have been selected during evolution.

Thus my colleagues and I have borrowed a Sanskrit philosophical term, *vasana*, to describe this new type of social chemosignal. The word *vasana* derives from *vas*, meaning "to perfume," and is "an unconscious impression left on the mind" (McClintock, 2001). Note that this is a functional definition, referring to the effect of the social chemosignal, as do the term *odor* and *pheromone*. In time, the evidence from the social neurosciences in all four explanatory dimensions may converge, demonstrating that androstadienone is indeed a human pheromone. If so, it will introduce a new class of modulator pheromones to the literature. Meanwhile, the evidence to date clearly demonstrates that androstadienone is a vasana, which, without conscious detection, modulates human reactions to social interactions through its action on the nervous and endocrine systems.

More broadly, this discussion of pheromones and vasanas is an example calling for social neuroscientists to approach their research topics in all four dimensions of explanation (Goldin-Meadow et al., 2003). Each dimension is essential for a full explanation: multiple levels of organization, mechanistic and functional causes, time spans including the life span and evolution as well as the moment, and finally, both objective and subjective perspectives on dynamic interactions.

References

Goldin-Meadow, S., McClintock, M. K., & Wimsatt, W. A. (2004). Solving psychological problems in four dimensions: Heuristics for the social and biological sciences. Manuscript in preparation.

Jacob, S., Kinnunen, L., Metz, J., Cooper, M., & McClintock, M. K. (2001). Sustained Human Chemosignal Unconsciously Alters Brain Function. *NeuroReport, 12,* 2391–2394.

Jacob, S., Spencer, N. A., Bullivant, S. B., Sellergren, S. A., Mennella, J., & McClintock, M. K. (2004). Effects of breastfeeding chemosignals on the human menstrual cycle. *Human Reproduction, 19(2),* 1–8.

Jacob, S., Zelano, B., Hayreh, D. J. S., & McClintock, M. K. (2002). Assessing putative human pheromones. In C. Rouby, B. Schall, A. Holley, D. Dubois, R. Gervais (Eds.), *Olfaction, taste and cognition.* (pp. 178–195). Cambridge: Cambridge University Press.

McClintock, M. K. (1998). Whither menstrual synchrony? *Annual Review of Sexual Research, 9,* 77–95.

McClintock, M. K. (2000). Human pheromones: Primers, releasers, signalers or modulators? In K. Wallen & J. E. Schneider (Eds.), *Reproduction in context: Social and environmental influences on reproductive physiology and behavior* (pp. 355–420). Cambridge, MA: MIT Press.

McClintock, M. K. (2001). Pheromones and vasanas: The functions of social chemosignals. In J. A. French, A. C. Kamil, & D. W. Leger (Eds.), *Evolutionary psychology and motivation nebraska symposium* (Vol. 48, pp. 75–112). Lincoln: University of Nebraska Press.

McClintock, M. K. (2002). Pheromones, odors and vasanas: The neuroendocrinology of social chemosignals in humans and animals. In D. Pfaff et al. (Eds.), *Hormones, brain and behavior* (Vol. 1, pp. 797–870). San Diego: Academic Press.

Shinohara, K., Morofushi, M., & Kimura, F. (1999). Effects of human pheromones on pulsatile luteinizing hormone secretions. *Neuroscience Research Supplement, 23,* S233.

Stern, K., & McClintock, M. K. (1998). Regulation of ovulation by human pheromones. *Nature, 392*, 177–179.

Weller, A., & Weller, L. (2002). Menstrual synchrony can be assessed, inherent cycle variability notwithstanding: Commentary on Schank (2001). *Journal of Comparative and Physiological Psychology, 116*, 316–318.

Weller, L., Weller, A., Koresh-Kamin, H., & Ben-Shoshan, R. (1999). Menstrual synchrony in a sample of working women. *Psychoneuroendocrinology, 24*, 449–459.

Zehr, J. L., Gans, S. E., & McClintock, M. K. (2001). Variation in reproductive traits is associated with short anogenital distance in female rats. *Developmental Psychobiology, 38*, 229–238.

7 Affective Style: Causes and Consequences

Richard J. Davidson

Among the most salient features of emotion is the extraordinary variability across individuals in how they respond to emotionally significant events and people in their environment. Indeed, such individual differences in emotional responding are the qualities most commonly used to characterize other people; they are at the core of personality, and at the root of issues of vulnerability and resilience underlying a broad spectrum of psychiatric, and some physical, disorders. Historically, the study of individual differences in affect-related processes and personality has been based on self-report, interviews, or projective measures. Although the corpus of data generated via these methods has been useful in mapping the terrain of this general area, it is clear that such methods, and the conceptual frameworks on which they are based, are incomplete at best and potentially misleading. Our neighboring subdiscipline of cognitive psychology several decades ago moved away from self-report measures as method for understanding mechanism. There was general agreement among cognitive psychologists that the inferences subjects make about their cognitive processes are limited and that, though they generally have access to the products of cognitive computations, they have little access to the processes that lead to those products. Thus, for example, we are all aware of the fact that we generate grammatical sentences, but we have little introspective access into the specific processes and computations required to produce such complex cognitive function. In the domain of affective functioning, I believe we stand today at a historical threshold as important as that crossed by the study of cognitive processes 30–40 years ago. Even though the vast majority of the extant research on emotion has relied on self-report measures, there is growing recognition of the need to move beyond such measures, particularly in the effort to understand the mechanisms giving rise to individual differences in emotional reactivity.

Affective style generally refers to a broad range of individual differences in specific features of emotional responding. This essay will consider the types of parameters that define specific features of affective style. Measurement issues loom large in this literature, and the essay will showcase the multiple modalities that have been used to make inferences about the causes and consequences of affective style, providing examples of research designed to examine the proximal neural causes and peripheral biological consequences of individual differences in affective style. Finally, the essay will consider plasticity in the neural circuitry subserving affective style, a topic that has broad implications for the treatment of psychopathology and for the promotion of healthy social and emotional functioning.

The Nature and Measurement of Affective Style

In several recent publications, I have defined *affective style* as valence-specific features of emotional reactivity and affective responding and suggested that the term be used to denote a broad range of individual differences in different parameters of emotional reactivity (Davidson, 1998a, 2000). The choice of the word *style* in defining this construct is meant to imply that these are individual differences that are relatively consistent over time and across situations. "Consistent," however, does not mean "immutable to change." There are likely developmental differences in sensitivity to change with certain developmental periods being "sensitive periods," where the organism is more susceptible to change. From the perspective adopted in this essay, such sensitive periods are likely subserved by developmental differences in neuroplasticity (Davidson, Jackson, & Kalin, 2000), a theme to which I will return at the end of this essay.

I have previously suggested that five specific parameters of affective style can be objectively measured: (1) the threshold to respond; (2) the magnitude of the response; (3) the rise time to the peak of the response; (4) the recovery function of the response; and (5) the duration of the response. These parameters of affective style refer to changes in various physiological systems that reflect emotion and can be assessed in these multiple systems in response to stimuli, events or people that have affective significance. The extent to which there is coherence across different physiological systems in these parameters of affective style is an unanswered question and will likely vary with the specific systems in question and the specific nature of the stimuli or events used as a challenge.

Parameters (3–5) of affective style all refer to different aspects of affective chronometry or the time course of emotional responding. My colleagues and I have proposed that time course variables are particularly germane to understanding individual differences that may reflect vulnerability to psychopathology:

certain forms of mood and anxiety disorders may be specifically associated with a failure to turn off a response sufficiently quickly, an abnormally early onset of the response that may then result in a bypassing of normal regulatory constraints, or both. All five specific parameters of affective style described above jointly govern in a complex fashion the dispositional mood and other reportable characteristics that are commonly reflected in self-report measures of affect-related personality constructs. This section will summarize findings from my laboratory on relations between individual differences in both prefrontal and amygdala function and measures that reflect affective style.

In a lengthy series of studies, my colleagues and I first established that, when subjects are presented with certain types of positive or negative emotional stimuli, the asymmetric activation of brain electrical activity in prefrontal scalp regions systematically changes (see, for example, Davidson & Tomarken, 1989). Basic observations using measures of brain electrical activity have been conceptually replicated with positron-emission tomography, providing considerably better spatial resolution (Sutton et al., 1997). On the basis of both our empirical efforts and a theoretical framework derived in part from a synthesis of a wide range of information that included data from comparative ethology, behavioral neurology, and neuroscience, we predicted that approach-related positive affect would be specifically associated with activation of left prefrontal regions, and withdrawal-related negative affect, with activation of right prefrontal regions (see, for example, Davidson, Ekman, Saron, Senulis, & Friesen, 1990). In a number of those early studies, we noticed that the valence-dependent changes in brain electrical activity appeared to be superimposed upon individual differences in the direction and magnitude of these prefrontal electrical asymmetries. Moreover, the variation across individuals was consistently larger than any change we observed within an individual between conditions. Furthermore, we found that a simple resting baseline measure of activation asymmetry in brain electrical measures from prefrontal scalp regions correlated highly with the average brain electrical asymmetry across the various stimulation conditions we presented. Thus we reasoned that we could use a simple measure of resting baseline signal to capture individual differences in tonic levels of asymmetric prefrontal activation. We predicted that such baseline individual differences would be related to certain features of valence-specific affective responding.

During our initial explorations of this phenomenon, we needed to determine whether baseline electrophysiological measures of prefrontal asymmetry were reliable and stable over time and thus could be used as a traitlike measure. Tomarken, Davidson, Wheeler, and Doss (1992) recorded baseline brain electrical activity from 90 normal subjects on two occasions separately by approximately 3 weeks. At each testing session, brain activity was recorded during eight 1-minute trials. Our focus was on power in the alpha band (8–13 Hz), though we extracted power in all frequency bands (for methodological discussion, see Davidson, J. P. Chapman, L. P. Chapman, & Henriques, 1990; Davidson, Jackson, & Kalin, 2000). We computed coefficient alpha as a measure of internal consistency reliability from the data for each session. The coefficient alphas were quite high, with all values exceeding .85, indicating that the electrophysiological measures of asymmetric activation indeed showed excellent internal consistency reliability. The test-retest reliability was adequate, with intraclass correlations ranging from .65

to .75 depending on the specific sites and methods of analysis. Our study demonstrated that measures of activation asymmetry based on power in the alpha band from prefrontal scalp electrodes show both high internal consistency reliability and acceptable test-retest reliability and can therefore be considered a traitlike index. Similar findings have recently been obtained by Hagemann, Naumann, Thayer, and Bartussek (2002).

On the basis of our prior data and theory, we reasoned that extreme left and extreme right frontally activated subjects would show systematic differences in dispositional positive and negative affect. We administered the trait version of the Positive and Negative Affect Scales (PANAS) to examine this question and found that the left-frontally activated subjects reported more positive and less negative affect than their right-frontally activated counterparts (Tomarken, Davidson, Wheeler, & Doss, 1992). More recently with Sutton (Sutton & Davidson, 1997), I showed that scores on self-report measures designed to operationalize Gray's concepts, the Behavioral Inhibition Scale (BIS) and the Behavioral Activation Scale (BAS), were even more strongly predicted by electrophysiological measures of prefrontal asymmetry than were scores on the PANAS. Subjects with greater left-sided prefrontal activation reported more relative BAS to BIS activity than subjects exhibiting more right-sided prefrontal activation (cf. Davidson, 1998b).

Sutton and I also predicted that our measures of prefrontal asymmetry would be related to reactivity to experimental elicitors of emotion. The model that my colleagues and I have developed over the past several years (for background, see Davidson, 1992, 1995, 1998a) features individual differences in prefrontal activation asymmetry as a reflection of a diathesis which modulates reactivity to emotionally significant events. It predicts that individuals who differ in prefrontal asymmetry should respond differently to an elicitor of positive or negative emotion, even when baseline mood is partialed out. We (Wheeler, Davidson, & Tomarken, 1993; see also Tomarken, Davidson, & Henriques, 1990) performed an experiment to examine this question. We presented short film clips designed to elicit positive or negative emotion. Brain electrical activity was recorded prior to the presentation of the film clips; subjects completed scales that were designed to reflect their mood at baseline. Just after the clips were presented, they were asked to rate their emotional experience during the preceding film clip. We found that individual differences in prefrontal asymmetry predicted the emotional response to the films even after measures of baseline mood were statistically removed. Those individuals with more left-sided prefrontal activation at baseline reported more positive affect to the positive film clips, whereas those with more right-sided prefrontal activation reported more negative affect to the negative film clips. These findings support the idea that individual differences in electrophysiological measures of prefrontal activation asymmetry mark some aspect of vulnerability to positive and negative emotion elicitors. That such relations were obtained following the statistical removal of baseline mood indicates that any difference between left- and right-frontally activated subjects in baseline mood cannot account for the prediction of film-elicited emotion effects that were observed.

The nomological network of associations I have thus far described have all involved relations between measures of individual differences in brain electrical indices of prefrontal activation asymmetry and self-report of mood. Although these associations have been novel and important in helping us to understand how asymmetries in prefrontal activation may contribute to features of affective style, they suffer from some of limitations noted at the outset concerning the utility of self-report data about emotion. In addition to the types of studies described, we have been amassing a number of findings relating individual differences in asymmetric prefrontal activation to peripheral biological measures that likely reflect the downstream consequences of such central circuitry. Some of these studies have been conducted with rhesus monkeys, who exhibit very similar variation to that seen in humans in affective style. The two types of peripheral measures we have most extensively examined include measures of the hypothalamic-pituitary-adrenal system (HPA; mostly cortisol) as well as measures of immune function (see, for example, Kalin, Larson, Shelton, & Davidson, 1998; Kalin, Shelton, & Davidson, 2000; Buss et al., 2003; Davidson, Coe, Dolski, & Donzeila, 1999). These studies establish an important link between individual differences in the central circuitry of emotion and downstream peripheral biological changes that may play important roles in both mental and physical health.

Although clearly suggesting that activation asymmetries in prefrontal cortex somehow are associated with individual differences in emotional reactivity and peripheral biological processes that may reflect such differences in emotional reactivity, the studies do not provide any further clues concerning a mechanistic account of how such differences may be produced. In regard to the more mechanistic issues of emotion regulation, my colleagues and I have proposed that one important function of specific territories of the prefrontal cortex and adjacent anterior cingulate cortex is to modulate activation in certain subcortical targets of emotional processing such as the amygdala. We have conceptualized emotion regulation as involving both automatic and voluntary components (see Davidson, Putnam, & Larson, 2000; Davidson, Jackson, & Kalin, 2000). Using brain electrical measures of individual differences in prefrontal activation asymmetry and emotion-modulated startle to examine the time course of emotional reactivity, we have found that those individuals with greater relative left-sided prefrontal activation at baseline are better able to downregulate negative affect as inferred from the attenuation of startle magnitude following the offset of a negative stimulus (Jackson et al., 2003). We know that there are anatomical connections between certain regions of prefrontal cortex and the amygdala through which this kind of inhibitory signal could be mediated. Using functional magnetic resonance imaging (fMRI) measures, we have also begun to show that instructions to voluntarily regulate negative affect do indeed produce measurable systematic variations of signal magnitude in the amygdala (Schaefer et al., 2002).

Plasticity and Affective Style

The circuitry that underlies emotion regulation, in particular, the amygdala and prefrontal cortex, has been a target of intensive study of plasticity (for thorough discussion, see Davidson, Jackson, & Kalin, 2000). In a series of elegant studies in rodents, Meaney and his colleagues (see Meaney, essay 1, this volume) have demonstrated that an early environmental manipulation in the rat's frequency of maternal licking and grooming and arched-back nursing, produces a cascade of biological changes in the offspring that shape the central circuitry of emotion and consequently, alter the animal's behavioral and biological responsivity to stress. In other research, Meaney and colleagues have reported that that rats exposed to high–licking and grooming mothers exhibited a permanent increase in concentrations of receptors for glucocorticoids in both the hippocampus and the prefrontal cortex (see Meaney, essay 1, this volume). All of these changes induced by early maternal licking and grooming and related behavior involve alterations in circuitry crucial to emotion and emotion regulation. In more recent work, researchers have found that enriched environmental experience results in large-scale increases in neurogenesis in the hippocampus in adult animals, suggesting that the environmental effects are not restricted to early life events.

These findings in animals raise the possibility that similar effects may transpire in humans. There are clearly short-term changes in brain activation that are observed during voluntary emotion regulation, as noted above. Whether repeated practice in techniques of emotion regulation lead to more enduring changes in patterns of brain activation is a question that has not yet been answered. There is limited evidence that cognitive behavioral therapy for certain disorders (e.g., obsessive compulsive disorder) produces changes in regional brain activity that are comparable to those produced by medication. What is absent are data on plastic changes in the brain that might be produced by the practice of methods specifically designed to increase positive affect, such as meditation. In a recent study, we (Davidson et al., 2003) examined changes in anterior activation asymmetry produced by an 8-week course in stress reduction based on mindfulness meditation. We compared subjects randomly assigned to a mediation group or a wait-list control group on measures of baseline brain electrical asymmetry (in addition to other measures) before and after the 8-week intervention. The intervention consisted of one 2.5-hour class per week, along with a request that subjects practice 45 minutes per day. We found that subjects in the meditation group showed an increase in left-sided anterior activation, whereas subjects in the wait-list control group showed a change in the opposite direction. We also administered an influenza vaccine following the completion of the 8-week course to subjects in both the meditation and control groups. Remarkably, we found that subjects in the meditation group showed a larger increase in antibody titers to the influenza vaccine than the controls did, and that the magnitude of shift toward more left-sided anterior activation was associated with a larger increase in antibody titers.

Summary and Conclusions

This essay provides a brief introduction to the study of affective style from a neuroscience perspective. Progress in this domain has been facilitated by the use a broad array of methods that include traditional psychophysiological measures, hormonal and immune measures, and neuroimaging techniques. It is clear from the early progress in this research domain that our traditional concepts of individual differences in emotion-related personality functioning will soon give way to more refined analysis of more specific parameters of affective style that can be measured objectively and that are rooted in well-understood neural systems. We have seen how, despite findings of stability in measures of asymmetric prefrontal function, we can expect at least some plasticity in this circuitry and that certain forms of training may facilitate change in salubrious directions. We can expect that this progress in research on affective style will have important benefits for assessing and intervening in a wide range of disorders and will provide important clues for new methods that might promote resilience.

Acknowledgments

The research reported in this essay was generously supported by grants MH43454, MH40747, P50-MH52354, and P50-MH61083 from the National Institute of Mental Health, by grants from the Research Network on Mind-Body Interaction of the John D. and Catherine T. MacArthur Foundation, and by assistance from the University of Wisconsin. I am deeply indebted to the many students and collaborators associated with the Laboratory for Affective Neuroscience and the W. M. Keck Laboratory for Functional Brain Imaging and Behavior who made this work possible.

References

Buss, K. A., Malmstadt, J. R., Dolski, I., Kalin, N. H., Goldsmith, H. H., & Davidson, R. J. (2003). Right frontal brain activity, cortisol, and withdrawal behavior in 6-month-old infants. *Behavioral Neuroscience*, *117*, 11–20.

Davidson, R. J. (1992). Emotion and affective style: Hemispheric substrates. *Psychological Science*, *3*, 39–43.

Davidson, R. J. (1995). Cerebral asymmetry, emotion and affective style. In R. J. Davidson, and K. Hugdahl (Eds.), *Brain asymmetry* (pp. 361–387). Cambridge, MA: MIT Press.

Davidson, R. J. (1998a). Affective style and affective disorders: Perspectives from affective neuroscience. *Cognition and Emotion*, *12*, 307–320.

Davidson, R. J. (1998b). Anterior electrophysiological asymmetries, emotion and depression: Conceptual and methodological conundrums. *Psychophysiology*, *35*(5), 607–614.

Davidson, R. J. (2000). Affective style, psychopathology, and resilience: Brain mechanisms and plasticity. *American Psychologist, 55*, 1196–1214.

Davidson, R. J., Chapman, J. P., Chapman, L. P., & Henriques, J. B. (1990). Asymmetrical brain electrical activity discriminates between psychometrically matched verbal and spatial cognitive tasks. *Psychophysiology, 27*, 238–543.

Davidson, R. J., Coe, C. C., Dolski, I., & Donzella, B. (1999). Individual differences in prefrontal activation asymmetry predict natural killer cell activity at rest and in response to challenge. *Brain, Behavior, and Immunity, 13*, 93–108.

Davidson, R. J., Ekman, P., Saron, C., Senulis, J., & Friesen, W. V. (1990). Approach/withdrawal and cerebral asymmetry: Emotional expression and brain physiology, I. *Journal of Personality and Social Psychology, 58*, 330–341.

Davidson, R. J., Jackson, D. C., & Kalin, N. H. (2000). Emotion, plasticity, context, and regulation: perspectives from affective neuroscience. *Psychological Bulletin, 126*, 890–909.

Davidson, R. J., Jackson, D., & Larson, C. (2000). Human electroencephalography. In J. T. Cacioppo, G. Bernston, and L. Tassinary (Eds.), *Principles of psychophysiology* (2nd ed.; pp. 27–52). New York: Cambridge University Press.

Davidson, R. J., Kabat-Zinn, J., Schumacher J., Rosenkranz, M., Muller, D., Santorelli, S. F., et al. (2003). Alterations in brain and immune function produced by mindfulness meditation. *Psychosomatic Medicine, 65*, 564–570.

Davidson, R. J., Putnam, K. M., & Larson, C. L. (2000). Dysfunction in the neural circuitry of Emotion Regulation: A possible prelude to violence. *Science, 289*, 591–594.

Davidson, R. J., & Tomarken, A. J. (1989). Laterality and emotion: An electrophysiological approach. In F. Boller, and J. Grafman (Eds.), *Handbook of neuropsychology* (Vol. 3., pp. 419–441). Amsterdam: Elsevier.

Hagemann, D., Naumann, E., Thager, J. F., & Bartussek, D. (2002). Does resting electroencephalograph asymmetry reflect a trait? An application of latent state-trait theory. *Journal of Personality and Social Psychology, 82,* 619–641.

Jackson, D. C., Mueller, C. J., Dolski, I., Dalton, K. M., Nitschke, J. B., Urry, H. L., et al. (2003). Now you feel it, now you don't: Frontal brain electrical asymmetry and individual differences in emotion regulation. *Psychological Science, 14,* 612–617.

Kalin, N. H., Larson, C. L., Shelton, S. E., & Davidson, R. J. (1998). Asymmetric frontal brain activity, cortisol, and behavior associated with fearful temperament in rhesus monkeys. *Behavioral Neuroscience, 112,* 286–292.

Kalin, N. H., Shelton, S. E., & Davidson, R. J. (2000). Cerebrospinal fluid corticotropin-releasing hormone levels are elevated in monkeys with patterns of brain activity associated with fearful temperament. *Biological Psychiatry, 47,* 579–585.

Schaefer, S. M., Jackson, D. C., Davidson, R. J., Aguirre, G. K., Kimberg, D. Y., & Thompson-Schill, S. L. (2002). Modulation of amygdalar activity by the conscious regulation of negative emotion. *Journal of Cognitive Neuroscience, 14,* 913–921.

Sutton, S. K., & Davidson, R. J. (1997). Prefrontal brain asymmetry: A biological substrate of the behavioral approach and inhibition systems. *Psychological Science, 8,* 204–210.

Sutton, S. K., Ward, R. T., Larson, C. L., Holden, J. E., Perlman, S. B., & Davidson, R. J. (1997). Asymmetry in prefrontal glucose metabolism during appetitive and aversive emotional states: An FDG-PET study. *Psychophysiology, 34,* S89.

Tomarken, A. J., Davidson, R. J., & Henriques, J. B. (1990). Resting frontal activation asymmetry predicts emotional reactivity to film clips. *Journal of Personality and Social Psychology, 59,* 791–801.

Tomarken, A. J., Davidson, R. J., Wheeler, R. E., & Doss, R. C. (1992). Individual differences in anterior brain asymmetry and fundamental dimensions of emotion. *Journal of Personality and Social Psychology, 62,* 676–687.

Tomarken, A. J., Davidson, R. J., Wheeler, R. E., & Kinney, L. (1992). Psychometric properties of resting anterior EEG asymmetry: Temporal stability and internal consistency. *Psychophysiology, 29,* 576–592.

Wheeler, R. E., Davidson, R. J., & Tomarken, A. J. (1993). Frontal brain asymmetry and emotional reactivity: A biological substrate of affective style. *Psychophysiology, 30,* 82–89.

8 When Memory Sins

Daniel L. Schacter

The emerging field of social neuroscience is in some respects similar to, and in others different from, the somewhat older and more established field known as cognitive neuroscience. The similarities lie in the general approach and goals of the two enterprises: both cognitive neuroscience and social neuroscience seek to link levels of analysis—psychological and biological—by using complementary methodologies, including cognitive and behavioral analyses, studies of brain-damaged patients, and neuroimaging techniques such as functional magnetic resonance imaging (fMRI). The main difference concerns the content domain of the two approaches: cognitive neuroscientists focus on such processes as attention, language, memory, and thought, irrespective of their social contexts, whereas social neuroscientists attempt to elucidate the social contexts and implications of these and other basic psychological processes.

Because both approaches rely on a similar cross-level linking analysis, it is reasonable to expect that they should inform one another. In this chapter, I will describe a cognitive neuroscience approach to human memory that has recently begun to address issues and questions of interest to social neuroscientists. Specifically, I will focus on research that is examining errors and illusions of memory. Because they can provide insight into the basic architecture and functioning of memory systems, at both the psychological and neural levels of analysis, memory's imperfections are of great theoretical interest. I will first outline seven categories or types of memory imperfections, which I have called the "seven sins of memory" (Schacter, 1999, 2001a), by analogy to the seven deadly sins. I then focus on how a cognitive neuroscience approach is beginning to illuminate the neural correlates and foundations of the memory sins, and in so doing touch on some implications for social neuroscience.

The Seven Sins of Memory: A Brief Overview

Scientists have long known that memory is subject to forgetting and distortion, but there have been few systematic attempts to classify and organize our knowledge of memory's errors. The proposal that memory's imperfections can be classified into seven sins (Schacter, 1999, 2001a) represents one such attempt.

The first three of the seven sins, different types of forgetting, can be thought of as sins of omission. The first sin, *transience*, refers to the fact that memories tend to become decreasingly accessible over time, a pervasive feature of memory first documented in the laboratory by Ebbinghaus (1885/1964) and central to all theories of remembering and forgetting. The second sin, *absentmindedness*, refers to lapses of attention that result in forgetting to do things. We all experience this kind of irritating, everyday forgetfulness when we cannot recall where we placed our keys or eyeglasses moments ago. The third sin, *blocking*, refers to information that has not faded out of memory but is temporarily inaccessible. The most common example of blocking is probably the "tip of the tongue" experience, where we temporarily cannot retrieve a name or word that, nevertheless, we are certain that we know (e.g., Schwartz, 1999; Maril, Wagner, & Schacter, 2001).

The next three sins, in which memory is present, but wrong, can be viewed as sins of commission. *Misattribution*, the fourth of our seven sins, occurs when we remember that something happened to us and attribute the memory to an incorrect source. For example, having imagined carrying out a task, we may mistakenly come to believe that we actually did it (Johnson, Hashtroudi, & Lindsay, 1993). The fifth sin, *suggestibility*, refers to implanted memories that are produced by leading questions or suggestions. Dramatic examples of suggestibility have been documented in which individuals seemingly recover vivid, even traumatic memories of events that never happened (for review, see McNally, 2003; Schacter, 2001a). The sixth (and final distortion-related) sin, *bias*, refers to the ways in which our current knowledge and beliefs can skew our memories. Numerous studies have shown that what we know, believe, and feel in the present can powerfully influence and distort the past (Ross & Wilson, 2000). Finally, the seventh sin, *persistence*, refers to unwanted memories of difficult or even traumatic experiences that people cannot forget. Persisting memories can, in extreme cases, permanently color how we view the present, past, and future, such as the intrusive memories sometimes experienced by war veterans or survivors of sexual assault (McNally, 2003).

Cognitive neuroscience has focused intensively on a few of the sins, and very little on others. For example, it has long been known that damage to the inner or medial aspects of the temporal lobe, including the hippocampus, produces a profound amnesic syndrome, which is characterized by an inability to retain new memories that can later be consciously recollected (e.g., Squire, 1992). A great deal of effort has been expended in attempting to understand this extreme form of transience. Similarly, a good deal of research has recently focused on understanding persisting emotional memories that appear to depend heavily on the amygdala and related structures (e.g., LeDoux, 1996). In contrast, next to nothing is known about the cognitive neuroscience of suggestibility and bias. In this essay, I will briefly consider two of the seven sins that we have examined in our laboratory: transience and misattribution. We are beginning to make strides in understanding these sins, and some of the lessons learned have implications for issues of concern to social neuroscience.

Transience

Cognitive neuroscience approaches to transience, as noted earlier, have focused intensively on amnesic patients with medial temporal lobe damage, who exhibit transience to an extreme degree, often forgetting experiences as fast as they occur. During recent years, studies using fMRI in healthy volunteers have begun to provide complementary insights into an important source of transience: initial encoding of information into memory. It has long been known from cognitive research that semantic or elaborative encoding typically results in more robust retention than does nonsemantic or shallow encoding. Event-related functional magnetic resonance imaging (fMRI) procedures make it possible to track encoding processes on a trial-by-trial basis. Responses can be sorted later, according to whether an item is remembered or forgotten (for review and discussion, see Paller & Wagner, 2002).

A study from our laboratory (Wagner, Schacter, Rotte, Koutstaal, Maril, Dale, et al., 1998) used event-related fMRI to determine whether responses to individual words during encoding predict subsequent remembering and forgetting of those words. Participants viewed a long list of words and decided whether each word was abstract or concrete, followed by a non-scanned recognition test. Comparison of high-confidence hits (i.e., "old" responses to studied words accompanied by high confidence) with misses ("new" responses to studied words) revealed, at the time of encoding, significant activation in the left medial temporal lobe, as well as in several left prefrontal regions. Thus level of activity in these regions during encoding was related to whether an individual word was later remembered or forgotten. Another fMRI study from our laboratory (Wagner et al., 1998) indicated that these prefrontal and medial temporal activations are linked to increased semantic encoding (compared with non-semantic encoding). Numerous studies carried out during the past few years have produced similar findings (Paller & Wagner, 2002).

These results suggest that transience is more likely to occur when specific prefrontal and medial temporal regions are not strongly engaged at the time of encoding than when they are. The results have also stimulated research that is of more direct relevance to social neuroscience. Consider, for instance, the well-known self-reference effect: information that is encoded in relation to ourselves is usually better remembered than other types of semantic information (for review, see Symons & Johnson, 1997). Building on the aforementioned encoding studies, Kelley and colleagues (2002) scanned subjects while they judged whether a series of trait adjectives (e.g., *honest*, *friendly*) did or did not describe themselves (self-referent encoding) or a familiar other person (George Bush; semantic encoding without self-referent encoding). In addition, these conditions were compared with a nonsemantic encoding condition in which participants judged whether words appeared in upper- or lowercase. Consistent with earlier work, semantic versus nonsemantic encoding activated an area in the lower left prefrontal cortex. Self-referent encoding, however, activated a different frontal region, the medial prefrontal cortex. These results suggest that self-referent and semantic encoding differ qualitatively; self-referent encoding does not appear to be simply a stronger type of semantic encoding that results in increased activation in the same brain region.

Misattribution

As noted earlier, misattribution errors occur when we attribute a memory of something imagined or false to something actual or true, or a memory of something actual or true to the wrong source. One of the most intensively studied forms of misattribution is known as false recognition: when people mistakenly claim that a novel item has been experienced previously. We have been attempting to gain insight into the neural bases of misattribution errors through neuropsychological studies of patients with specific brain lesions, and neuroimaging studies of healthy populations. For instance, we conducted a series of experiments exploring false recognition in a patient with a lesion to the right frontal lobe who exhibited strikingly elevated levels of false recognition (Curran, Schacter, Norman, & Galluccio, 1997; Schacter, Curran, Gallucio, Milberg, & Bates, 1996). The patient, referred to by the initials B.G., falsely recognized words, sounds, pictures, and other materials at an extremely high rate, far greater than that of matched control subjects. B.G. appeared to have difficulty monitoring familiarity signals, which he frequently misattributed to a specific prior encounter that never occurred. In a subsequent fMRI study that examined memory for previously encountered words, where participants were required to recollect both an item and its source (in this experiment, the kind of encoding task that subjects had performed on the item), we found that right frontal regions are especially active when healthy subjects needed to closely monitor small differences in item familiarity (Dobbins, Rice, Wagner, & Schacter, 2003). Taken together, these complementary lines of research indicate that right frontal regions play an important role in retrieval processes that are central to understanding misattribution errors.

We have also used neuropsychological and neuroimaging approaches to examine the contribution of medial temporal lobe regions to misattribution errors that are observed when people falsely recognize novel items due to semantic or perceptual similarity with previously studied items. For example, Roediger and McDermott (1995) modified and extended a procedure developed initially by Deese (1959), in which subjects hear lists of associated words (e.g., *candy, sour, sugar, bitter, good, taste, tooth*). All of the words are strong associates of a nonpresented critical lure word (e.g., *sweet*). Roediger and McDermott reported striking levels of false recognition (e.g., 80 percent), accompanied by high confidence, to the critical lure words. Participants appear to misattribute the strong sense of familiarity or recollection elicited by the critical lure to having heard or seen the critical lure words during the study phase of the experiment.

To examine the role of the medial temporal lobes in this type of misattribution, we tested amnesic patients; as discussed earlier, these patients have damage to the medial temporal lobe and related structures. Several studies from our laboratory using the Deese–Roediger and McDermott procedure have revealed that amnesic patients exhibit lower levels of false recognition to critical lure words than do healthy controls (e.g., Schacter, Verfaellie, & Pradere, 1996; Verfaellie, Schacter, & Cook, 2002). Similarly, we have found that amnesics exhibit lower levels of false recognition to lure items that are perceptually related to large numbers of previously studied shapes (Koutstaal, Schacter, Verfaellie, Brenner, & Jackson, 1999) and objects (Koutstaal, Verfaellie, & Schacter, 2001).

Neuroimaging studies provide further evidence concerning the role of the medial temporal lobe in false recognition of semantic associates. We scanned subjects as they made true and false recognition judgments concerning previously studied words, associatively related critical lures, and unrelated lure words that were not associatively linked to any previously studied lists. Compared with the unrelated lure control condition, the hippocampus showed significant—and indistinguishable—levels of activation during both true and false recognition (Cabeza, Rao, Wagner, Mayer, & Schacter, 2001; see also Schacter, Reiman, et al., 1996; Schacter, Buckner, Koutstaal, Dale, & Rosen, 1997). Taken together, the neuropsychological and neuroimaging evidence suggests that regions within the medial temporal lobe, including the hippocampus, are involving in storing or retrieving associative information, or both, that contributes to the false recognition of critical lures.

Recent work in our laboratory, led by Jason Mitchell, has used some of the insights discussed above concerning encoding and transience to explore a different type of misattribution, one of considerable interest to social neuroscience: the illusion of truth. This illusion occurs when exposure to a statement increases subsequent confidence that the statement is true, even when people are cued that the statement is false (e.g., Gilbert, Krull, & Malone, 1990). Subjects appear to misattribute familiarity with a previously exposed statement to increased truth value, but the illusion of truth can be reduced when subjects are able to specifically recollect that a statement was cued false (Begg, Anas, & Farinacci, 1992), In Mitchell's study (Mitchell, Dodson, & Schacter, 2003), we scanned participants while they viewed statements that were cued as true or false (neutral items were also included). The key finding was that regions in the prefrontal cortex and medial temporal lobe, whose activation during encoding in previous studies was associated with successful subsequent recollection, showed greater activation at encoding for those statements on which subjects were later able to avoid the illusory truth effect than for those statements that showed illusory truth. These observations provide converging neural evidence for the cognitive hypothesis that false statements can be rejected, and the illusion of truth thus reduced, when participants recollect specific details of what they encoded about a particular statement.

Concluding Comments and Future Directions

A key strength of the cognitive neuroscience approach to memory involves reliance on converging evidence from independent sources, such as the neuropsychological and neuroimaging studies reviewed here that are beginning to illuminate several of the memory sins. This same approach will no doubt will be a feature of social neuroscience. Such an approach might provide not only strong tests of theoretical hypotheses, but also fresh perspectives on classical problems of social psychology. As an example of this latter possibility, consider a study by Lieberman, Ochsner, Gilbert, and Schacter (2001) that examined the role of conscious, explicit memory in the phenomenon of cognitive dissonance—the psychological discomfort that occurs when behavior conflicts with beliefs. Social psychologists have for the most part assumed that the experience of dissonance requires an ability to recall the behavior that produced conflict in the first place. If so, then people who are unable to consciously recollect recent experiences, such as amnesic patients, should not exhibit signs of cognitive dissonance. Using a paradigm that created dissonance by requiring participants to choose between two art prints that they liked, we found that both amnesics and controls reduced dissonance by later inflating how much they liked the chosen print relative to the bypassed print—even though the amnesic patients had no conscious memory for making the choice that produced the dissonance. Such findings highlight that conscious memory may play a lesser role in dissonance phenomena than was previously suspected. They also provide insights that are relevant to the memory sin of bias because dissonance reduction involves resculpting the past to fit the present. This type of social neuroscience approach can illuminate both classical issues of social psychology and the imperfections and achievements of memory.

Acknowledgments

Preparation of this chapter was supported by grant AG08441 from the National Institute on Aging and by grant NS60941 from the National Institute of Mental Health.

References

Begg, I. M., Anas, A., & Farinacci, S. (1992). Dissociation of processes in belief: Source recollection, statement familiarity, and the illusion of truth. *Journal of Experimental Psychology: General, 121*, 446–458.

Cabeza, R., Rao, S. M., Wagner, A. D., Mayer, A. R., & Schacter, D. L. (2001). Can medial temporal lobe regions distinguish true from false? An event-related fMRI study of veridical and illusory recognition memory. *Proceedings of the National Academy of Sciences, U.S.A., 98*, 4805–4810.

Curran, T., Schacter, D. L., Norman, K. A., & Galluccio, L. (1997). False recognition after a right frontal lobe infarction: Memory for general and specific information. *Neuropsychologia, 35*, 1035–1049.

Deese, J. (1959). On the prediction of occurrence of particular verbal intrusions in immediate recall. *Journal of Experimental Psychology, 58*, 17–22.

Dobbins, I. G., Rice, H. J., Wagner, A. D., & Schacter, D. L. (2003). Memory orientation and success: Separable neurocognitive components underlying episodic recognition. *Neuropsychologia, 41*, 318–333.

Ebbinghaus, H. (1885/1964). *Memory: A contribution to experimental psychology.* New York: Dover.

Gilbert, D. T., Krull, D. S., & Malone, P. S. (1990). Unbelieving the unbelievable: Some problems in the rejection of false information. *Journal of Personality and Social Psychology, 59*, 601–613.

Johnson, M. K., Hashtroudi, S., & Lindsay, D. S. (1993). Source monitoring. *Psychological Bulletin, 114*, 3–28.

Kelley, W. M., Macrae, C. N., Wyland, C. L., Caglar, S., Inati, S., & Heatherton, T. F. (2002). Finding the self?: An event-related fMRI study. *Journal of Cognitive Neuroscience, 14*, 785–794.

Koutstaal, W., Schacter, D. L., Verfaellie, M., Brenner, C., & Jackson, E. M. (1999). Perceptually-based false recognition of novel objects in amnesia: Effects of category size and similarity to prototype. *Cognitive Neuropsychology, 16*, 317–342.

Koutstaal, W., Verfaellie, M., & Schacter, D. L. (2001). Recognizing identical vs. similar categorically related common objects: Further evidence for degraded gist-representations in amnesia. *Neuropsychology, 15*, 268–289.

LeDoux, J. E. (1996). *The emotional brain*. New York: Simon and Schuster.

Lieberman, M. D., Ochsner, K. N., Gilbert, D. T., & Schacter, D. L. (2001). Do amnesics exhibit cognitive dissonance reduction? The role of explicit memory and attention in attitude change. *Psychological Science, 12*, 135–140.

Maril, A. Wagner, A. D., & Schacter, D. L. (2001). On the tip of the tongue: An event-related fMRI study of retrieval failure and cognitive conflict. *Neuron, 31*, 653–660.

McNally, R. J. (2003). Remembering trauma. Cambridge, MA: Harvard University Press.

Mitchell, J. P., Dodson, C. S., & Schacter, D. L. (2003). Counteracting misattribution: An event-related fMRI study of illusory truth. Manuscript submitted for publication.

Paller, K. A., & Wagner, A. D. (2002). Observing the transformation of experience into memory. *Trends in Cognitive Science, 6*, 93–102.

Roediger, H. L., III, & McDermott K. B. (1995). Creating false memories: Remembering words not presented in lists. *Journal of Experimental Psychology: Learning, Memory, and Cognition, 21*, 803–814.

Ross, M., & Wilson, A. E. (2000). Constructing and appraising past selves. In D. L. Schacter & E. Scarry (Eds.), *Memory, brain, and belief* (pp. 231–258). Cambridge, MA: Harvard University Press.

Schacter, D. L. (1999). The seven sins of memory: Insights from psychology and cognitive neuroscience. *American Psychologist, 54*, 182–203.

Schacter, D. L. (2001a). *The seven sins of memory: How the mind forgets and remembers.* Boston: Houghton Mifflin.

Schacter, D. L. (2001b). Suppression of unwanted memories: Repression revisited? *Lancet, 357,* 1724–1725.

Schacter, D. L., Buckner, R. L., Koutstaal, W., Dale, A., & Rosen, B. (1997). Late onset of anterior prefrontal activity during true and false recognition: An event-related fMRI study. *NeuroImage, 6,* 259–269.

Schacter, D. L., Curran, T., Galluccio, L., Milberg, W., & Bates, J. (1996). False recognition and the right frontal lobe: A case study. *Neuropsychologia, 34,* 793–808.

Schacter, D. L., Reiman, E., Curran, T., Sheng Yun, L., Bandy, D., McDermott, K. B., et al. (1996). Neuroanatomical correlates of veridical and illusory recognition memory: Evidence from positron-emission tomography. *Neuron, 17,* 1–20.

Schacter, D. L., Verfaellie, M., & Pradere, D. (1996). The neuropsychology of memory illusions: False recall and recognition in amnesic patients. *Journal of Memory and Language, 35,* 319–334.

Schwartz, B. L. (1999). Sparkling at the end of the tongue: The etiology of tip-of-the-tongue phenomenology. *Psychonomic Bulletin and Review, 6,* 379–393.

Squire, L. R. (1992). Memory and the hippocampus: A synthesis from findings with rats, monkeys, and humans. *Psychological Review, 99,* 195–231.

Symons, C. S., & Johnson, B. T. (1997). The self-reference effect in memory: A meta-analysis. *Psychological Bulletin, 121,* 371–394.

Verfaellie, M., Schacter, D. L., & Cook, S. P. (2002). The effect of retrieval instructions on false recognition: Exploring the nature of the gist memory impairment in amnesia. *Neuropsychologia, 40,* 2360–2368.

Wagner, A. D., Schacter, D. L., Rotte, M., Koutstaal, W., Maril, A., Dale, A. M., et al. (1998). Building memories: Remembering and forgetting of verbal experiences as predicted by brain activity. *Science, 281,* 1188–1190.

9 Multilevel Analyses and Reductionism: Why Social Psychologists Should Care about Neuroscience and Vice Versa

Gary G. Berntson and John T. Cacioppo

Social and biological explanations of behavior have often been considered to offer distinct, or even incompatible, alternative accounts. This was not always the case, however. The Darwinian revolution attracted broad attention and generated infectious enthusiasm for understanding the biological bases of social behavior (for review, see Berntson & Cacioppo, 2000b). Unfortunately, attention faded and enthusiasm soon dampened, due in large part to the vacuous application of simplistic and untestable biological causes (e.g., instincts) to explain all social behavior. By the middle of the twentieth century, a deep schism and enduring mutual suspicion had arisen between social psychologists and psychobiologists; their respective professional "evolutions" began to diverge.

Psychobiologists emphasized physiological processes, neural substrates, and production mechanisms for behavior, often eschewing mentalist and functionalist theories, or considering them subject to reductionism. In contrast, social psychologists emphasized multivariate systems, situational influences, and practical applications, and strongly rejected reductionism. Consequently, these psychological subdisciplines progressed along two diverging trajectories that yielded what some regarded as an unbridgeable rift between social and biological approaches (Scott, 1991). Minimally, these divergences resulted in vastly different subject samples, research traditions, methodologies, and theoretical perspectives.

As unbridgeable as this rift may have seemed at one time, several major developments are helping to allay the once profound mutual suspicion between social psychology and psychobiology. One is the increasing recognition that psychobiological perspectives can offer important insights into complex social problems, such as aggression or drug addition, and that social processes are not only consequences of, but also impact on, psychobiological operations. In addition, recent methodological developments, such as functional brain imaging, now offer a powerful research armamentarium that supports meaningful studies of brain systems and social processes. Finally, the utility of interdisciplinary, multilevel approaches and analyses in understanding complex systems has contributed to the emergence of social neuroscience. This discipline is grounded in the recognition of the inherent links across levels of organization and analysis and in the fundamental construct of reductionism, as opposed to substitutionism. *Reductionism* embraces the ability to relate one level of organization (e.g., the social) to another (e.g., the hormonal), but recognizes that causal links between levels go both ways, and that lower levels of analysis can never entirely replace or substitute for higher-level analyses. The opposing construct of *substitutionism* holds that one level of analysis (generally a higher) can be replaced or supplanted by another level (generally a lower), and the goal of science is the pursuit of explanations at the lowest possible level of analysis. In contrast to this view, and in agreement with reductionism as defined here, emerging perspectives in neuroscience, and especially the new field of social neuroscience, emphasize the complementing nature of social and biological levels of analysis and how each can contribute to an understanding of complex behaviors and the mind.

Social Neuroscience

We are pleased to have contributed to the emergence of the field of social neuroscience (Cacioppo & Berntson, 1992; Cacioppo et al., 2002; Ochsner & Lieberman, 2001). Although there has been a rich history of research linking social and biological perspectives, it has been only recently that the field has developed a coherent presence and a clear identity. Indeed, not until 1992 was the term *social neuroscience* introduced as a descriptive label for this field (Cacioppo & Berntson, 1992).

Before starting our collaborative program in 1989, we had both established programs entailing multiple levels of analysis, which extended from the social to the psychophysiological level (Cacioppo); and from the psychophysiological to the neural level (Berntson). We shared a recognition of the importance of cross-level analyses, and the merging of our research and perspectives afforded the groundwork for a collaborative effort extending from the macro (social) to the micro (neural) levels of organization and analysis. Two early findings from our collaborative effort illustrate the utility of multilevel analyses. One deals with the impact of social factors on autonomic cardiovascular control and health, and the other on the potential impact of autonomic states on higher social and cognitive processes.

Multiple Levels of Organization: Top-Down Influences of Social Factors

The autonomic nervous system has traditionally been viewed as a homeostatic mechanism for maintaining a stable internal state. This perspective emerged from early research in the Walter Cannon era that focused on the peripheral components of the autonomic nervous system and the homeostatic reflex mechanisms of the lower brain stem that regulate these peripheral pathways. It is now clear that higher neural systems also impact autonomic control, and often in a fashion that does not comport with a simple homeostatic model, but rather reflects an *allodynamic* process through which more flexible and adaptable patterns of control can be achieved (see Berntson, Cacioppo, & Quigley, 1991; Berntson & Cacioppo, 2000a). An illustration of this comes from studies of autonomic responses to stressors.

In accord with the homeostatic reflex model of autonomic control, the sympathetic and parasympathetic nervous systems, which often have opposing effects, have been traditionally viewed as reciprocally controlled. When one branch is activated, the other is inhibited, and thus both branches act synergistically to achieve the same outcome. An increase in blood pressure, for example, results in a reflexive activation of parasympathetic outflow and a parallel reduction in sympathetic outflow. The increased parasympathetic activity results in a slowing of the heart, and the decreased sympathetic activity yields a further reduction in heart rate as well as a relaxation of vascular walls and consequent vasodilation, all of which oppose the blood pressure perturbation. The brainstem neural circuitry and neurophysiological mechanisms that underlie this reflexive hemostatic control have been fairly well characterized.

Findings from our studies of stressors confirm this reciprocal mode of autonomic control with changes in blood pressure. We employed single and dual pharmacological blockades of the autonomic branches to examine sympathetic and parasympathetic responses to the physiologic stress of standing up from a sitting position (orthostatic stress), which reduces blood pressure and triggers a homeostatic reflex response. Results revealed an increase in heart rate attributable to an increase in sympathetic control, together with a decrease in parasympathetic control. In accord with the reciprocal model of control, the individual responses of the two branches of the autonomic nervous system were highly (negatively) correlated. There is ample support for the historical focus on the reciprocal mode of autonomic control, but this model is incomplete. Although it may apply to many lower reflexes, higher neurobehavioral systems (e.g., those mediating social cognition) can have more diverse influences on autonomic control.

In the same blockade study, we also determined autonomic responses to social-cognitive stressors (e.g., speech stress). At a group level, the social stressor also yielded an increase in heart rate, comparable to the orthostatic stressor, which was associated with an overall sympathetic activation and parasympathetic withdrawal. In contrast to the orthostatic stressor, however, there were considerable individual differences in the pattern of response, and hence there was no correlation between the activities of the autonomic branches. Rather, some subjects showed a rather selective and reliable increase in sympathetic control, others a selective decrease in parasympathetic control, and still others showed various combinations of these responses.

These and similar findings, in a social context, have mandated an expansion of a major physiological model of autonomic control.

Autonomic states can no longer be viewed as lying along a single continuum from sympathetic to parasympathetic dominance, but rather can assume a broader range of functional states described by an autonomic space. This autonomic space is described by a bivariate representation, in which sympathetic activity is indicated along one axis and parasympathetic activity along an orthogonal axis. This autonomic space model can thus incorporate all possible combinations of sympathetic and parasympathetic activities, as well as response patterns characterized by independent, reciprocal, or even coactive changes in the two autonomic branches (Berntson & Cacioppo, 2000a). These are important findings because individual patterns of response may reflect distinct psychological states and have differential implications for health. These considerations point to the need for more sophisticated conceptualizations of stress.

Although orthostatic stress yielded highly concordant responses in all subjects, there were individual differences in the pattern of autonomic response to psychological stress, and these differences (but not the former) were predictive of neuroendocrine and immunological status. Specifically, sympathetic cardiac reactivity, but not parasympathetic cardiac reactivity or overall heart rate change, was predictive of hypothalarnic pituitary-adrenocortical response and (inversely) of the immunological response to vaccine (Cacioppo, 1994; Cacioppo et al., 1995). Similarly, the clinical outcome after myocardial infarction appears to be a function in part of the specific pattern of cardiac autonomic control, with sympathetic control being a risk factor and parasympathetic control having a protective effect.

The impact of social factors on autonomic and neuroendocrine control has also become apparent through our recent research on loneliness. Personal ties are a ubiquitous part of life, serving important social, psychological, and behavioral functions across the life span. Moreover, it is becoming increasingly apparent that positive social relationships are important for physical and psychological well-being.

Epidemiological research has found that social isolation is a major risk factor for morbidity and mortality from widely varying causes, including cardiovascular diseases, even after statistically controlling for other known risk factors. Moreover, experimental research in animals has further confirmed that social stressors can contribute to cardiovascular disease in primates. Although there are several routes by which social factors may impact health, one likely candidate is a unique pattern of autonomic and neuroendocrine control that appears to characterize loneliness (Cacioppo et al., 2002).

Importantly, in the absence of measures and analyses at the social or macro level, the effects of loneliness on health would be obscure, and individual differences attributable to these factors would simply appear as error variance in medical models.

Multiple Levels of Organization: Bottom-Up Influences

The social neuroscience perspective entails not only considerations of how social factors impact biology, but also how social processes are realized in the brain, and how biological factors may impact these mechanisms. There is now an expanding literature on brain systems that mediate social processes, ranging from neurophysiological and neurochemical studies in animals to brain-imaging studies in humans. Our focus in this area, however, has been decidedly more cross-level. That is, we have asked how lower-level factors, such as autonomic states, might impact higher-level cognitive and social processes (Cacioppo, Berntson, & Klein, 1992; Berntson, Sarter, & Cacioppo, 2003). This has been a topic of interest since William James articulated what is now referred to as "the James-Lange theory of emotion," in which emotions are considered to be the perceptual consequences of somatovisceral feedback.

Although the strong form of this concept is no longer tenable, it is increasingly clear that bottom-up, ascending visceral influences can importantly modulate higher-level processes such as memory, emotion, and cognition (Cacioppo et al., 1992; Berntson et al., 2003). Indeed, the specific neural pathways mediating these effects are beginning to be elucidated. Parallel noradrenergic and cholinergic routes extend from visceral sensory receiving areas in the nucleus of the tractus solitarius, directly and indirectly to the locus coeruleus, the amygdala, the basal forebrain cholinergic system, and the cerebral cortex. These ascending systems have been repreatedly implicated in neurobehavioral processes. Damasio and colleagues (see Damasio, 1994), for example, offer neuropsychological evidence that the amygdalocortical (especially medial prefrontal) circuits are involved in guiding behavior based on environmental and somatovisceral feedback. Additionally, the ascending basal forebrain cholinergic system is an important regulator of cerebral cortical function and has been implicated in cortical activation, attention, anxiety, and cognition (Berntson, Sarter, & Cacioppo, 1998, in press). These ascending regulators of cortical state strongly impact the highest-level cortical processes that underlie the unique characterstics, accomplishments, and sociocultural heritage of the human race.

The concept of an ascending regulatory system in the brain has been with us since the work in the mid-twentieth century on the ascending reticular activating system and arousal. The arousal construct promised to link cognitive function with neural mechanisms and had broad impact on psychology and social psychology. This construct died a merciful death, as it became apparent from the behavioral perspective that arousal is neither monolithic nor continuous. It also became apparent from the neuroscientific perspective that what was thought to be a rather homogenous and nonspecific ascending arousal system in fact comprises multiple, neurochemically and neuroanatomically differentiated and functionally specific pathways. This is a particularly exciting set of developments; work in this area is beginning to clarify conceptual complexities and empirical inconsistencies in the "arousal" literature and to more critically elucidate brain-behavior relations. It also illustrates how behavioral and neural analyses can yield converging insights and constrain or inform concepts and theories across levels of analysis.

Summary

There is much to be gained by multilevel analyses in general, and social neuroscience approaches in particular. A rational reductionistic approach, one that eschews substitutionism, can benefit each level of analysis. All behavior is biological, but biological reductionism does not yield a simple, singular, or satisfactory explanation for complex behaviors, and micro forms of representation do not provide the only or even necessarily the best level of analysis for understanding human behavior. Micro or neural perspectives and analyses may offer tremendous insights on macro or social processes. On the other hand, macro constructs of the social sciences provide an efficient means of organizing and understanding highly complex activity without needing to specify each individual action of the simplest components (Cacioppo, Berntson, Sheridan, & McClintock, 2000). Moreover, macro constructs serve to define issues and topics that serve as the subject matter for micro approaches and often represent the dependent variables that allow evaluation of theories and inferences derived from micro approaches. It is the mutual interaction, calibration, and orchestration across levels of analysis that will represent the next important wave of developments in the social sciences.

Although descending and ascending neural influences generally act synergistically, there are discernible effects and interactions from processes at distinct levels of the neuraxis. Primitive protective responses to aversive stimuli, for example, are organized at the level of the spinal cord, as is apparent in flexor (pain) withdrawal reflexes that can be seen even after spinal transaction (Berntson, Boysen, & Cacioppo, 1993). These primitive protective reactions are expanded and embellished at higher levels of the nervous system. The evolutionary development of higher neural systems, such as the limbic system, endowed organisms with an expanded behavioral repertoire, including escape reactions, aggressive responses, and even the ability to anticipate and avoid aversive encounters (Berntson et al., 1993). Evolution not only endowed us with primitive, lower-level adaptive reactions, but it sculpted the remarkable information processing capacities of the highest levels of the brain. Thus neurobehavioral mechanisms are not localized to a single level of organization within the brain, but rather are represented at multiple levels of the nervous system. At progressively higher (more rostral) levels of organization (spinal, brain stem, limbic, cortical regions) there is a general expansion in the range and relational complexity of contextual controls and in the breadth and flexibility of discriminative and adaptive responses (Berntson et al., 1993).

Adaptive flexibility of higher-level systems has costs, given the finite information-processing capacity of neural circuits (Berntson et al., 1993). Greater flexibility implies a less rigid relationship between inputs and outputs, a greater range of information that must be processed, and a slower serial-like mode of processing. Consequently, the evolutionary layering of higher processing levels onto lower substrates has adaptive advantage in that lower and more efficient processing levels may continue to be utilized and may be sufficient in some circumstances (Berntson et al., 1998). Higher neurobehavioral processes, however, can come to suppress or bypass pain withdrawal reflexes (Boysen, Berntson, Hannan, & Cacioppo, 1996). A person unwittingly touching a hot flame normally experiences a rapid, autonomic, reflexive withdrawal from the painful fire. If, however, the person hears a child on the other side of a wall of flames, this defensive reflex can be overridden by higher-level motivations, with the person most likely looking for a doorway or passage not engulfed by flames or donning fire-retardant covering (e.g., a wet blanket) before challenging the fire to retrieve the child. Both animal models and a variety of non-invasive recordings in humans (event-related brain potentials, functional magnetic resonance imaging) have proved useful in exploring the more complex interactive processes across levels of the neuraxis, and new methods and approaches are continually emerging. This is an especially exciting effort—multilevel approaches will be central in understanding the brain and behavior.

Acknowledgments

Preparation of this essay was supported by grant (HL 54428) from the National Institute of Heart, Lung and Blood and by grant (BCS-0086314) from the National Science Foundation.

References

Berntson, G. G., Boysen, S. T., & Cacioppo, J. T. (1993). Neurobehavioral organization and the cardinal principle of evaluative bivalence. *Annals of the New York Academy of Science, 702*, 75–102.

Berntson, G. G., & Cacioppo, J. T. (2000a). From homeostasis to allodynamic regulation. In J. T. Cacioppo, L. G. Tassinary, & G. G. Berntson (Eds.), *Handbook of psychophysiology* (pp. 459–481). Cambridge: Cambridge University Press.

Berntson, G. G., & Cacioppo, J. T. (2000b). Psychobiology and social psychology: Past, present, and future. *Personality and Social Psychology Review, 4*, 3–15.

Berntson, G. G., & Cacioppo, J. T. (2003). A contemporary perspective on multilevel analyses and social neuroscience. In F. Kessel, P. L. Rosenfield, & N. Anderson. (Eds.), *Expanding the boundaries of health and social science: Case studies in interdisciplinary innovation* (pp. 18–40). New York: Oxford University Press.

Berntson, G. G., Cacioppo, J. T., & Quigley, K. S. (1991). Autonomic determinism: The modes of autonomic control, the doctrine of autonomic space, and the laws of autonomic constraint. *Psychological Review, 98*, 459–487.

Berntson, G. G., Sarter, M., & Cacioppo, J. T. (1998). Anxiety and cardiovascular reactivity: The basal forebrain cholinergic link. *Behavioural Brain Research, 94,* 225–248.

Berntson, G. G., Sarter, M., & Cacioppo, J. T. (2003). Ascending visceral regulation of cortical affective information processing. *European Journal of Neuroscience, 18,* 2103–2109.

Boysen, S. T., Berntson, G. G., Hannan, M. B., & Cacioppo, J. T. (1996). Quantity-based interference and symbolic representations in chimpanzees (*Pan troglodytes*). *Journal of Experimental Psychology: Animal Behavior Processes, 22,* 76–86.

Cacioppo, J. T. (1994). Social neuroscience: autonomic, neuroendocrine, and immune responses to stress. *Psychophysiology, 31,* 113–128.

Cacioppo, J. T. (2002). Social neuroscience: Understanding the pieces fosters understanding the whole and vice versa. *American Psychologist, 57,* 819–830.

Cacioppo, J. T., & Berntson, G. G. (1992). Social psychological contributions to the decade of the brain: Doctrine of multilevel analysis. *American Psychologist, 47,* 1019–1028.

Cacioppo, J. T., Berntson, G. G., & Klein, D. J. (1992). What is an emotion? The role of somatovisceral afference, with special emphasis on somatovisceral "illusions." *Review of Personality and Social Psychology, 14,* 63–98.

Cacioppo, J. T., Berntson, G. G., Sheridan, J. F., & McClintock, M. K. (2000). Multi-level integrative analyses of human behavior: Social neuroscience and the complementing nature of social and biological approaches. *Psychological Bulletin, 126,* 829–843.

Cacioppo, J. T., Hawkley, L. C., Crawford, L. E., Ernst, J. M., Burleson, M. H., Kowalewski, R. B., et al. (2002). Loneliness and health: Potential mechanisms. *Psychosomatic Medicine, 64,* 407–417.

Cacioppo, J. T., Malarkey, W. B., Kiecolt-Glaser, J. K., Uchino, B. N., Sgoutas-Emch, S. A., Sheridan, J. F., et al. (1995). Heterogeneity in neuroendocrine and immune responses to brief psychological stressors as a function of autonomic cardiac activation. *Psychosomatic Medicine, 57,* 154–164.

Damasio, A. R. (1994). *Descartes' error: Emotion, reason, and the human brain.* New York: Grosset/Putnam.

Ochsner, K. N., & Lieberman, M. D. (2001). The emergence of social cognitive neuroscience. *American Psychologist, 56,* 717–734.

Scott, T. R. (1991). A personal view of the future of psychology departments. *American Psychologist, 46,* 975–976.

10   Emotion, Social Cognition, and the Human Brain

Ralph Adolphs

The subject matter of our work has concerned how the brain processes emotional and social information. One guiding hypothesis has been that most social behavior involves emotion—a relationship that is reflected in the shared brain structures that subserve these two domains. There is also no shortage of real-life examples demonstrating their correlation. When someone smiles at us, speaks to us in a particular tone of voice, or when other people look at us, these sensory signals both evoke emotions within us and serve as social communication. The key tasks our brains face in everyday life is how to generate reliable social knowledge and how best to guide our own social behavior, given what is often an overwhelmingly complex array of sometimes very subtle sensory cues (Adolphs, 2003).

In some respects, social perception is no different from perception in general. One way of thinking about how we generate knowledge from sensory input is to view the mind as a collection of processes that construct a model of the world—the social world, in our case. In other ways, social perception differs from perception in general: social information is generally more complex, less predictable, and more interactive. For example, our close scrutiny of, say, a table will not change the visual appearance of the table; but our close scrutiny of another person certainly will (if they notice that they are being scrutinized). This interactive nature of social cognition makes some unique demands on the information processing required, and has resulted in brain systems that appear relatively specialized. Neuroscientists have found evidence for structures in the brain that are more important for processing social than nonsocial stimuli. This initial and robust finding in turn has motivated a series of further questions that we are now pursuing. What features of stimuli trigger such social brain processes? How specialized is the function of particular brain structures—if there are some relatively specialized to process social stimuli, might there be some that are specialized to process only certain subtypes of social stimuli? And how do multiple brain structures work together so that their concerted action yields adaptive behavior? Taken together, these questions aim to understand humans as a social species from the point of view of cognitive neuroscience.

The contributions my laboratory has made to these questions have been driven by particular approaches of method and of theory. Every method in isolation has its limitations, and a strength of many studies in social cognitive neuroscience is in the integration of data using multiple techniques. My colleagues and I have been using the lesion method in neurological patients, direct electrical recordings of brain activity in neurosurgical patients, functional imaging, studies of neuropsychiatric populations, and computational modeling. Most of our work has capitalized on the lesion method, pioneered at the University of Iowa by Antonio and Hanna Damasio (Damasio & Damasio, 1989), which tests hypotheses about the normal function of a brain structure by examining the impairments that result from focal damage to that structure. For instance, we hypothesized that the human amygdala would normally be important for recognizing fear from facial expressions. This hypothesis was supported by finding that selective amygdala damage impairs precisely this ability (Adolphs, Tranel, Damasio, & Damasio, 1994). Two critical components of the lesion method require thorough neuropsychological evaluation of all the subjects, provided by Daniel Tranel's neuropsychology clinic, and detailed neuroanatomical characterization from magnetic resonance scans of their brains, provided by Hanna Damasio's neuroimaging laboratory. Together, these components permit us to assign subjects to groups on the basis of the location of their lesion (e.g., amygdala-lesioned versus brain-damaged control), and to either match them or covary the groups for factors such as background IQ.

No less important than the technical resources available has been the theoretical framework for understanding social cognition. An overarching theme is that social knowledge is generated by the brain in a very creative way, rather than simply retrieved from storage in some sense. In particular, we use emotions, and their implementation as somatic states of the body, in order to reconstruct social information. This idea derives in part from Antonio Damasio's somatic marker hypothesis (Damasio, 1994). The idea also acknowledges current views on situated cognition—that cognition does not engage only the brain, but the body and the external environment as well. This picture of cognition sees stimuli as providing only a trigger to an elaborate, complex, and creative set of processes that generate knowledge and behavior. Those processes, while guided in large part by the brain, incorporate the structure and reactivity of the body and the external environment.

Lesion Studies

Earlier work by my colleagues and me documented a role for structures such as the amygdala (Adolphs et al., 1994) and right somatosensory cortices (Adolphs, Damasio, Tranel, Cooper, & Damasio, 2000) in the recognition of emotion from facial expressions. These findings suggested an information-processing architecture according to which perceptual representations of the features of faces and their configuration were linked to the generation of knowledge about the emotion that they signal via several parallel mechanisms. One mechanism, the one on which we had focused, was presumed to depend on the construction of a simulation, in the viewer, of aspects of the internal emotional state of the observed person. Roughly speaking, the idea was that the amygdala stored associations between faces and bodily emotional reactions, and could therefore be used to reenact components of the bodily emotional response when shown the facial expression. That is, seeing an emotional face literally triggered an emotional state in the viewer, an idea for which there is some experimental evidence, but about whose significance there is still disagreement.

The role for somatosensory cortices in emotion recognition was presumed to operate at a subsequent information-processing stage: a central representation of the emotional state triggered by the face. Our data, and other findings from functional imaging, additionally indicated that premotor cortices would be important, and for a similar reason: they would permit a representation of the motor patterns required to produce the emotional behaviors observed in the stimulus. These findings on emotion recognition fit nicely with a popular new account of action recognition, according to which observed actions are mapped onto the motor representations that would normally be engaged if one were producing the action oneself. Together, then, the important roles of the amygdala and somatosensory cortices supported the idea that the brain constructs social knowledge, at least in part, by simulating the emotional state of an observed person: we know how other people feel because we mirror their feelings.

As a further investigation of the generality of the mechanism, we have asked subjects to attribute emotions and personality traits to a variety of stimuli. In regard to faces, we found that the amygdala was important not only for recognizing emotions from facial expressions, but also for judging whether people's faces looked trustworthy or approachable (Adolphs, Tranel, & Damasio, 1998). Andrea Heberlein showed subjects various visual stimuli, such as point light displays and body postures, and assessed the social attributions they make from them. Amygdala, somatosensory, and premotor cortices were again revealed to be important, although there were interesting differences in the extent to which these structures contributed to different kinds of attributions (such as emotions versus personality traits). We also presented subjects with auditory stimuli, such as prosody and music, and again found evidence for a similar network of structures. Addressing the question of specificity posed above, we found evidence that the amygdala was most important for the recognition of emotion from faces, rather than from other kinds of stimuli. In one experiment that showed this clearly, subjects were presented with two sets of social scenes that conveyed various emotions: one set containing facial expressions of people, the other set identical except that the faces had been digitally erased. As one would expect, normal subjects were more accurate in recognizing the emotions shown in these scenes when they contained facial expressions. Surprisingly, subjects with amygdala damage showed the converse pattern: they were worse when the scenes contained faces, presumably because facial expressions were one cue in whose recognition they were disproportionately impaired (Adolphs & Tranel, 2003).

When these findings are taken together, we can think of the amygdala as implementing a particular process: the association of a sensory stimulus with an emotional state. That process, in turn, can be used in a variety of ways: for recognition of emotion from facial expressions, by triggering emotional states that permit simulation of what another person would feel like; for more complex social judgments about other people that also rely on the generation of an emotional state and a feeling about those people; and for other domains of cognition whose function is modulated by emotion, such as emotional memory. Of course, the amygdala is not the only structure that participates in these functions, and a current research direction is to more clearly specify the role of some of the other components.

Neurosurgical Studies

In interpreting data from cognitive neuroscience, we wish to be careful to avoid phrenological formulations. If, for instance, the amygdala is important, even necessary, for the recognition of certain emotions from faces, then the next question is: with what other structures does the amygdala participate in accomplishing this, and what are the processes implemented by each of these neural components? To explore this question in greater detail, we need to look to techniques other than the lesion method. Functional magnetic resonance imaging, event-related potential, and magneto-encephalographic (MRI, ERP and MEG) recordings can provide something like a movie of brain activation. There is another, much more precise technique, although its application is extremely rare. In collaboration with the neurosurgeon Matthew Howard at the University of Iowa, my colleagues and I have been recording intracranially from patients who have electrodes implanted for epilepsy monitoring. Because the electrodes are implanted for clinical reasons, we are limited in recording from whatever tissue needs to be monitored in order to localize epileptic foci.

This technique can localize information processing in the brain with high spatiotemporal resolution, and has the potential to answer a host of questions that our earlier findings had left open. For instance, we found that the prefrontal cortex (Kawasaki et al., 2001) and the amygdala (Oya, Kawasaki, Howard, & Adolphs, 2002) can provide a rapid, early evaluation of emotionally salient stimuli. Such an initial evaluation could then provide feedback modulation of visual cortices, as well as bias subsequent information processing by other brain regions. Such rapid brain responses probably reflect automatic evaluations that may also contribute to social stereotyping, and which would seem to precede any conscious recognition of the stimulus.

The lesion method also left open questions about the exact role of somatosensory cortices. I mentioned earlier that we think somatosensory cortices play a role in emotion recognition because they serve as the substrate for making available information about the emotional state associated with the stimulus. But somatosensory cortices comprise many different regions of the brain, such as primary somatosensory cortex, insular cortex (a visceral and pain-related sensory cortex) as well as multimodal cortices. Moreover, there is topographic organization within these different cortices. When we recognize a facial emotion by simulating the body state with which it is normally associated, do we use only the face representation of primary somatosensory cortex? That is, do we simulating only how it would feel to make the face we see? Or do we use more extensive regions, simulating the feeling of the body that would be associated with the expression shown on the face? To address this issue, my colleagues and I are recording from cortical grid and strip electrodes in the neurosurgical patients. Using many (e.g., 64) contacts concurrently over somatosensory cortex or within the insula permits us to undertake a detailed examination of neuronal activity within those regions during tasks that require emotion recognition.

Future Extensions

One important extension of the current studies is to combine the biological data with that from computational models. In one such study, done in collaboration with Gary Cottrell at the University of California, San Diego, we trained an artificial neural network to categorize facial expressions of emotion at an accuracy comparable to that of humans (Dailey, Cottrell, Padgett, & Adolphs, 2002). To our surprise, the model also showed numerous behaviors that in humans are typically attributed to semantic knowledge, such as categorical perception of the emotions and particular similarity relationships. For instance, people judge anger and disgust to be more similar than anger and surprise. This similarity obtains if they make judgments about facial expressions, sounds, stories, or just the words anger, disgust, surprise. Amazingly, the artificial neural network that classified faces solely on the basis of their geometric properties showed exactly the same similarity relationships. Presumably this indicates that, at least for facial expressions, social signals feature physical relationships that are at some level isomorphic with the semantic relationships of the concepts that they denote.

Another entirely different extension of our work has been to test neuropsychiatric populations. We are testing social cognition in individuals with autism, in collaboration with Joe Piven at the University of North Carolina, and in individuals with Williams syndrome, in collaboration with Ursula Bellugi at the Salk Institute. We are comparing the performances of these psychiatric subjects not only with those of adults who have focal brain lesions, but, because they are developmental disorders, also with children who have focal brain damage. Our goal is to find commonalities between the data from these different populations that may permit inferences about the neural dysfunctions underlying autism and Williams syndrome.

Conclusions

These are exciting times to be investigating the neuroscience of human emotion and social behavior. The tools available now make possible experiments that we could only have dreamed of in the past (actually, we could not even have dreamed of them), so much so that the data pouring in now outstrip the theories formulated to interpret them. Such interpretations, in turn, will require not only a broad knowledge of neuroscience and psychology, but also sophistication in philosophy of science and philosophy of mind in order to forge a framework that can connect multiple disciplines effectively.

And of course the study of emotion forces us to confront perhaps the most interesting and mysterious question of all: how does neuronal activity conspire to make us conscious of our emotional states and those of other people. It seems plausible that emotion, social cognition, and conscious experience will emerge as three aspects of the same problem, and that investigations of any one of them will permit a better understanding of the others.

Acknowledgments

The work summarized here could not have been done without the help of my colleagues at the University of Iowa. Antonio and Hanna Damasio, Daniel Tranel, Matthew Howard, Antoine Bechara, Thomas Grabowski, and Steven Anderson have all provided considerable resources to generate a highly collaborative setting. Numerous students and fellows, listed on our laboratory Web site, have done the bulk of the labor and continue now to push the studies in new directions of their own. Funding has been made possible by grants from the National Institutes of Health, the Sloan Foundation, the EJLB Foundation, the Klingenstein Fund, and the James S. McDonnell Foundation.

References

Adolphs, R. (2003). Investigating the cognitive neuroscience of social behavior. *Neuropsychologia*, *41*, 119–126.

Adolphs, R., Damasio, H., Tranel, D., Cooper, G., & Damasio, A. R. (2000). A role for somatosensory cortices in the visual recognition of emotions as revealed by three-dimensional lesion mapping. *Journal of Neuroscience*, *20*, 2683–2690.

Adolphs, R., & Tranel, D. (2003). Amygdala damage impairs recognition of emotion from scenes only when they contain facial expressions. *Neuropsychologia, 41,* 1281–1289.

Adolphs, R., Tranel, D., & Damasio, A. R. (1998). The Human amygdala in social judgment. *Nature, 393,* 470–474.

Adolphs, R., Tranel, D., Damasio, H., & Damasio, A. (1994). Impaired recognition of emotion in facial expressions following bilateral damage to the human amygdala. *Nature, 372,* 669–672.

Dailey, M. N., Cottrell, G. W., Padgett, C., & Adolphs, R. (2002). EMPATH: A neural network that categorizes facial expressions. *Journal of Cognitive Neuroscience, 14,* 1158–1173.

Damasio, A. R. (1994). *Descartes' error: Emotion, reason, and the human brain.* New York: Grosset/Putnam.

Damasio, H., & Damasio, A. R. (1989). *Lesion analysis in neuropsychology.* New York: Oxford University Press.

Kawasaki, H., Adolphs, R., Kaufman, O., Damasio, H., Damasio, A. R., Granner, M., et al. (2001). Single-unit responses to emotional visual stimuli recorded in human ventral prefrontal cortex. *Nature Neuroscience, 4,* 15–16.

Oya, H., Kawasaki, H., Howard, M. A., & Adolphs, R. (2002). Electrophysiological responses in the human amygdala discriminate emotion categories of complex visual stimuli. *Journal of Neuroscience, 22,* 9502–9512.

11   The Accidental Neuroscientist: Positive Resources, Stress Responses, and Course of Illness

Shelley E. Taylor

My early work as a health psychologist explored primarily the psychosocial ways in which people cope with illness rather than their biological concomitants. I became a social neuroscientist by accident, in order to pursue the directions in which my research was logically leading. My work has focused heavily on the adaptive aspects of positive illusions, namely, the exaggeratedly positive beliefs, such as optimism, personal control, and self-enhancement, that are protective of mental health. In a series of publications, my colleagues and I have reported evidence that positive and even somewhat inflated perceptions of oneself, the world, and the future are associated with criteria thought to be indicative of mental health. Some provocative initial findings led us to believe that these positive beliefs might foster physical health as well, and this possibility became the lure to enter the field of social neuroscience.

HIV and the Impact of Positive Beliefs on Health

Approximately fifteen years ago, Margaret Kemeny and I began a program of research in psychoneuroimmunology to explore the impact of positive beliefs on the progression of HIV. The advantages of using HIV infection as a disease model are several. Unlike other chronic diseases, HIV infection has meaningful indicators of disease progression, including CD4 t-lymphocytes and viral load, and thus the relation of potential predictors, including psychosocial variables, to disease course can be precisely charted. There are also known cofactors that can be reliably measured and controlled. Moreover, because the HIV-infected population is (unhappily) more youthful than is the case for other chronic diseases, the problems of comorbidity that are frequently seen in other chronically ill populations and that confound the assessment of psychological and biological covariation are less often encountered with HIV.

Through a series of controlled investigations, we were able to demonstrate that positive beliefs were protective against an adverse course of HIV. Specifically, in an investigation led by Geoffrey Reed, we studied men who had already been diagnosed with AIDS and found that those who realistically accepted their negative fate died 9 months earlier, on average, than those who believed that they could fight HIV and avoid what was then its inevitable downward course (Reed, Kemeny, Taylor, Wang, & Visscher, 1994). In a second study with men who were HIV-seropositive but asymptomatic (also led by Reed), we showed that AIDS-specific optimism was associated with a significantly lower likelihood of symptom development during a subsequent 2- to 3-year period (Reed, Kemeny, Taylor, & Visscher, 1999). Thus, positive beliefs appear to retard the progression of HIV at multiple points across the disease spectrum. In a third study, led by Julienne Bower, we discovered that having found meaning in an experience of bereavement was protective against declines in CD4 T-helper cells over a follow-up period in men who were HIV-seropositive (Bower, Kemeny, Taylor, & Fahey, 1998).

In the three studies, we controlled for a variety of potential cofactors that might explain those results, including age, time since diagnosis, psychological distress, fatigue, suicidal ideation, and use of AZT. None of these variables accounted for the effects. In addition, the men who believed that their downward course was inevitable did not practice poorer health behaviors, did not have lower levels of social support, and did not ignore their relevant symptoms or comply poorly with medical treatment, nor did the impact of positive and negative beliefs on course of disease appear to be mediated by psychological distress, depression, or other emotional states.

We speculated that positive beliefs might exert their protective effects on health by affecting stress systems, that is, sympathetic nervous system (SNS) and hypothalamic-pituitary-adrenal (HPA) axis responses to stress. Drawing on the assumption that the adverse impact of stressful events on bodily systems is cumulative—what McEwen has called "allostatic load" (see McEwen, chapter 4, this volume)—we suggested that people who hold positive beliefs about themselves, the world, and their future, including falsely positive beliefs, may be able to meet the inevitable stressors of life with more psychosocial resources (i.e., personal resources such as active coping strategies and interpersonal ones such as social support), thus reducing their stress responses and limiting the accumulating damage over time (Taylor, Kemeny, Reed, Bower, & Gruenewald, 2000). The studies of men with HIV infection, however, did not provide opportunities to examine this idea directly.

Positive Resources and Stress Responses

To address mechanisms whereby exaggeratedly positive beliefs may affect stress responses, my colleagues and I assessed the "positive illusions" of healthy participants through questionnaires and later brought them into a laboratory to go through challenging tasks consisting primarily of multiple mental arithmetic tasks. We measured baseline and stress-reactive heart rate, blood pressure, and cortisol levels. In these studies, we focused specifically on self-enhancement, one of the most common and widely documented positive illusions. Consistent with our hypothesis, we found that people who were more self-enhancing showed lower heart rate and blood pressure responses to stress, and their baseline cortisol levels were lower (although cortisol responses to the stress tasks did not show a similar pattern).

The question arises as to *why* positive beliefs may keep stress responses low. Possible mediators that our laboratory has explored include negative emotions, psychological adjustment, personal resources, or combinations of these. To date, the work has supported the role of positive resources as a mediator. That is, positive self-evaluations may confer resources, such as social support or the ability to cope with stressors actively, which provide a set of tools for dealing with a broad array of stressors. Those who have such tools may cope with stress with a lesser psychological and biological toll.

Overall, our findings to date suggest some important pathways by which positive beliefs and psychosocial resources may contribute to health. Specifically, these positive states may keep the responses of the sympathetic nervous system and of the hypothalamic-pituitary-adrenal axis to stress low, thereby retarding the accumulation of stress-related allostatic load (e.g., Taylor, Lerner, Sherman, Sage, & McDowell, 2003).

Stress Responses and Tending to Others

One of the most important psychosocial resources that people use for dealing with stressful events is social support. Long known to be protective against illness and associated with longer life, the specific mechanisms whereby social support produces these effects have nonetheless remained somewhat elusive. The approach that my colleagues and I have adopted has been to look at supportive relationships as a biopsychosocial stress reduction system with developmental antecedents and consequences. Specifically, our research efforts have focused on two questions. What are the effects of good and bad nurturing on health across the life span? And what is the impetus for providing nurturant behavior?

On the first point, our work has examined "risky families" and the effects of early family life on health across the life span. Our work was prompted, in part, by a growing literature suggesting that children who are exposed to maltreatment and abuse in childhood are at increased risk for a broad array of adverse health and mental health conditions throughout life. Unlike past research, however, our efforts have focused on "normal" family strain and conflict, namely, on irritable quarreling, cold or neglectful parenting, or both, which also appear to be associated with adverse consequences for emotional and social functioning and for health in offspring. In essence, our work is consistent with animal models developed by Meaney, Rosenblum, and others who have demonstrated the important effects of early nonnurturant maternal contact on an offspring's developing stress regulatory systems, especially the HPA axis, and on behaviors suggestive of poor emotion regulation (e.g., anxiety) and compromised social functioning (e.g., low rank, little grooming).

Like these animal researchers, we report evidence that risky family environments create vulnerabilities, interact with genetically based vulnerabilities, or both, in offspring, that produce disruptions in psychosocial and biological functioning (see Repetti, Taylor, & Seeman, 2002). Empirically, we have related a risky family environment to negative emotions and compromised social relationships, and to disruptions in stress-responsive biological regulatory systems, including autonomic and HPA axis functioning. For example, using a laboratory stress challenge paradigm, we found that people from risky family backgrounds were more likely to show an elevated, flat cortisol response to stress, stronger cardiovascular responses to the challenges (men only), and poorer self-rated health than people who had not experienced this early adverse family environment. Such a biobehavioral profile can lead to consequent cumulative risk for mental health disorders, major chronic diseases, and early mortality.

In this research, then, we have focused on the developmental antecedents of positive psychosocial resources and their effects on social, emotional, and biological regulatory systems and on health. From our investigations, we conclude that early family environment provides an important source of input to an individual's ability to develop psychosocial resources such as social relationships and emotion regulation skills; these resources, in turn, may partially mediate the impact of family environment on physiological and neuroendocrine responses to stress and, over the long-term, on health (Repetti et al., 2002; Taylor, Lerner, Sage, Lehman, & Seeman, in press).

The Tend-and-Befriend Model

The importance of maternal nurturance in the development of offspring biology and behavior is so evident in both animal and human research that the origins of tending cry out for attention. This has been the focus of our current work. My colleagues and I recently proposed a theory of female responses to stress as characterized by a pattern termed "tend-and-befriend" (Taylor, Klein et al., 2000). Specifically, we proposed that females' responses to stress are characterized, not as much by the fight-or-flight mechanisms so widely researched among males, but by patterns that involve caring for offspring under stressful circumstances and drawing on social groups to reduce joint vulnerability. This tend-and-befriend response may depend, in part, on the hormone oxytocin, long known to be implicated in nurturance, in affiliative responses to stress, and in lower responses of the sympathetic nervous system and hypothalamic-pituitary-adrenal axis to stress. Endogenous opioid peptides, which have similarly been tied to maternal and affiliative behavior and to lower stress responses, may also be implicated.

We are currently investigating these links, largely through the use of opportunistic paradigms. Oxytocin's effects are known to be enhanced by estrogen, and consequently, comparing groups of women who are naturally high or low in estrogen may lead to reliable differences in oxytocin-mediated effects on affiliation and SNS and HPA axis stress responses. Some of our work has enrolled older women who have elected (or not) to take hormone replacement therapy and thus vary reliably in their estrogen levels. Other research has enrolled young women whose estrogen levels covary reliably with the menstrual cycle. This work is still in progress, but our hypothesis is that the estrogen-enhanced effects of oxytocin that is released under stressful circumstances may lead to reduced SNS and HPA axis stress responses and to an increase in affiliative responses to stress.

Summary

The research program that my colleagues and I have undertaken has been devoted to understanding the positive resources that people bring to stressful circumstances that enable them to combat stress more effectively and keep its biological and psychosocial toll in check. By making use of a broad array of paradigms, including the disease model of progressive HIV infection in our early studies, laboratory stress tasks for observing the antecedents of exaggerated stress responses, and opportunistic paradigms such as hormone replacement therapy or natural fluctuations in the menstrual cycle to examine the effect of estrogen and oxytocin on social responses to stress, we have been able to move closer to an overall portrait of the regulatory functions that psychosocial resources may play in the development and maintenance of mental and physical health.

Acknowledgments

Preparation of this essay was supported by grant BCS-9905157 from the National Science Foundation and by grant MH 56880-05 from the National Institute of Mental Health.

References

Bower, J. E., Kemeny, M. E., Taylor, S. E., & Fahey, J. L. (1998). Cognitive processing, discovery of meaning, CD4 decline, and AIDS-related mortality among bereaved HIV-seropositive men. *Journal of Consulting and Clinical Psychology, 66,* 979–986.

Reed, G. M., Kemeny, M. E., Taylor, S. E., & Visscher, B. R. (1999). Negative HIV-specific expectancies and AIDS-related bereavement as predictors of symptom onset in asymptomatic HIV-positive gay men. *Health Psychology, 18,* 354–363.

Reed, G. M., Kemeny, M. E., Taylor, S. E., Wang, H.-Y. J., & Visscher, B. R. (1994). "Realistic acceptance" as a predictor of decreased survival time in gay men with AIDS. *Health Psychology, 13,* 299–307.

Repetti, R. L., Taylor, S. E., & Seeman, T. E. (2002). Risky families: Family social environments and the mental and physical health of offspring. *Psychological Bulletin, 128,* 330–366.

Taylor, S. E., Kemeny, M. E., Reed, G. M., Bower, J. E., & Gruenewald, T. L. (2000). Psychological resources, positive illusions, and health. *American Psychologist, 55,* 99–109.

Taylor, S. E., Klein, L. C., Lewis, B. P., Gruenewald, T. L., Gurung, R. A. R., & Updegraff, J. A. (2000). Biobehavioral responses to stress in females: Tend-and-befriend, not fight-or-flight. *Psychological Review, 107,* 411–429.

Taylor, S. E., Lerner, J. S., Sage, R. M., Lehman, B. J., & Seeman, T. E. (in press). Early environment, emotions, responses to stress, and health. *Journal of Personality.*

Taylor, S. E., Lerner, J. S., Sherman, D. K., Sage, R. M., & McDowell, N. K. (2003). Are self-enhancing cognitions associated with healthy or unhealthy biological profiles? *Journal of Personality and Social Psychology, 85,* 605–615.

Contributors

Ralph Adolphs
Department of Neurology
University of Iowa
Iowa City, Iowa

Gary G. Berntson
Department of Psychology
Ohio State University
Columbus, Ohio

John T. Cacioppo
Department of Psychology
University of Chicago
Chicago, Illinois

C. Sue Carter
Department of Psychiatry
University of Illinois at
Chicago
Chicago, Illinois

Richard J. Davidson
Laboratory for Affective
Neuroscience
Department of Psychology
University of
Wisconsin–Madison
Madison, Wisconsin

Bruce S. McEwen
Laboratory of
Neuroendocrinology
The Rockefeller University
New York, New York

Michael J. Meaney
Douglas Hospital Research
Centre
Montreal, Quebec, Canada

Daniel L. Schacter
Department of Psychology
Harvard University
Cambridge, Massachusetts

Esther M. Sternberg
Integrative Neural Immune
Program
National Institute of Mental
Health
National Institutes of Health
Bethesda, Maryland

Stephen J. Suomi
Laboratory of Comparative
Ethology
National Institute of Child
Health and Human
Development
National Institutes of Health
Bethesda, Maryland

Shelley E. Taylor
Department of Psychology
University of California, Los
Angeles
Los Angeles, California

Index